Oxford Medical Publications

Nerve blocks in palliative care

Nerve blocks in palliative care

By

Fiona Hicks
Consultant in Palliative Medicine
Leeds Teaching Hospitals Trust
Leeds, UK

Karen H. Simpson
Consultant in Pain Medicine
Leeds Teaching Hospitals Trust
Leeds, UK

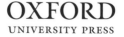
OXFORD
UNIVERSITY PRESS

OXFORD
UNIVERSITY PRESS

Great Clarendon Street, Oxford OX2 6DP

Oxford University Press is a department of the University of Oxford.
It furthers the University's objective of excellence in research, scholarship,
and education by publishing worldwide in

Oxford   New York

Auckland Bangkok Buenos Aires Cape Town Chennai
Dar es Salaam Delhi Hong Kong Istanbul Karachi Kolkata
Kuala Lumpur Madrid Melbourne Mexico City Mumbai Nairobi
São Paulo Shanghai Taipei Tokyo Toronto

Oxford is a registered trade mark of Oxford University Press
in the UK and in certain other countries

Published in the United States
by Oxford University Press Inc., New York

© Oxford University Press, 2004

A catalogue record for this title is available from the British Library

ISBN 0 19 8527039 (Pbk)

10 9 8 7 6 5 4 3 2 1

Typeset by Cepha Imaging Pvt. Ltd., Bangalore, India
Printed in Great Britain
on acid-free paper by
Biddles Ltd., Kings Lynn

Foreword

Pain is somehow everyone's business but often ends up being no-one's key concern. This book is written by two active clinicians who both work with patients in pain in palliative care. They approach the same patients from different angles – Dr Hicks from the palliative medicine physician's perspective and Dr Simpson as an anaesthetist interested in chronic pain and cancer pain.

The patient is at the heart of the matter – each clinician must ascertain how to ensure the patient's needs are known and then plans instigated to try to meet them. For the patient in pain, many of the psychological and social issues arising from their illness cannot be addressed. As anyone in pain knows, pain is all pervading. With control of pain comes the ability to tackle other issues, providing consciousness is not clouded by medication and the patient has the energy to think and ability communicate.

Rightly, this book takes the reader through the important process of assessment. Within the process the vulnerable patient must not be misled – the term pain 'control' is usually far more honest than the expectation of being 'pain-free'. The disease itself affects sensation, creating pain and other altered sensations – so even when pain is eased, the diseased part may never feel 'normal', or as it did before illness struck. Assessment is integrally linked to diagnosis of the underlying cause of the pain – accurate diagnosis then guides the management plan.

As the reader is taken through the pointers in assessment, it becomes clear that there are often several options therapeutically. The choice needs to be carefully matched to the individual patient. So knowledge of the options is crucial. The book covers simple blocks (Chapter 6), regional nerve blocks 'head to toe' (Chapter 7) and spinal analgesia (Chapter 8), taking the reader through the options so the clinician has realistic expectations of what can and cannot be done before discussing such possibilities with the vulnerable patient. The book does not provide enough detail to tell anyone how to do complex blocks or interventions; the specialist anaesthetist should be part of every regional palliative care service. But, in a very accessible way, the authors explain what is suitable for whom, what to expect and what the side-effects and complications are likely to be.

This book will be invaluable to palliative care specialists, medical, nursing and physiotherapy alike, as well as to the pain clinic anaesthetist and pain nurses. It promotes complementarity in team working and should allow more patients to access interventions that may be very helpful in pain control beyond currently prescribed opioids and co-analgesics. Lifelong learning is a duty for all – it is the only way patients will receive the care they deserve from their clinical services. This book will help the isolated practitioner as well as the trainer to realize the evolution of their own learning towards achieving better patient outcomes and less distress in those left behind after a patient has died.

Professor Ilora Finlay FRCP, FRCGP
(Baroness Finlay of Llandaff)

Preface

The incidence of cancer in adults continues to rise worldwide and despite significant advances in treatment many cancers remain incurable. Pain in cancer is one of the most feared symptoms and will affect most patients at some stage during their illness. The successful management of cancer pain is thus a priority for patients and their physicians. Similarly, many patients face a terminal illness other than cancer that requires palliative care. Studies in the UK have shown that pain is a significant problem in most patients during the last year of life irrespective of diagnosis although the nature of the pain has not been well described in patients with non-malignant disease.

There are many publications about cancer pain management and for approximately 90% of patients with cancer, pain can be managed successfully and simply, with acceptable side-effects, using oral analgesia alone. Similarly, the majority of patients with pain from progressive, non-malignant diseases gain adequate pain relief from oral analgesics. However, some patients with malignant or non-malignant disease may need more complex interventions ranging from simple nerve blocks to spinal analgesia. The term neuromodulation refers to techniques such as spinal drug delivery or spinal cord stimulation.

Consultants in pain management with expertise in the field of palliative care and with the time to become involved are scarce. There are large variations between and within regions. Palliative medicine physicians may not have experience of the full range of more interventional techniques that may benefit their patients. Many clinical nurse specialists in the field may not be fully conversant with all available treatment options; this is often true for other members of the multi-professional team. These factors may conspire to limit the choices available to patients with poorly controlled pain in the context of palliative care. They may not be offered relevant interventional treatments.

This book is designed to be a practical guide to nerve blocks and neuromodulation in adults and to help patients and professionals to make informed choices in pain management. We discuss appropriate patient selection and referral. Many patients may be frail with complex co-morbidity and the burdens and benefits of treatments must be carefully considered before embarking on any therapy. The timing of referral and intervention may be crucial. Patients must have pain that is likely to benefit from nerve blocks or neuromodulation, be fit enough to undergo the procedure and survive long enough to make it worthwhile. It is therefore important that the referring clinician is aware of what is involved in any procedure and able to provide appropriate aftercare. The window of opportunity is often quite small.

Many of the principles described may also apply to children with pain who need palliative care. However, children need special consideration that is beyond the scope of this book.

We hope that this book will help those in pain management and palliative care to consider all the options for analgesia. Such collaboration will optimize the care we provide for our patients.

F.H.

K.H.S.

Acknowledgements

Our thanks go to Dr David Barrow and Mr Eddy Richert for their technical support and encouragement.

Contents

Philosophy behind the use of interventional pain management techniques in palliative care

Pain is one of the most feared symptoms of cancer and other life-limiting diseases. Pain is the commonest reason for patients to present to doctors. The incidence of pain in cancer has been extensively studied[1–3] but there is less information about the incidence and nature of pain in patients with progressive non-malignant disease in the last few months or years of life.[4, 5] The majority of these 'palliative care' patients have their pain well managed using conventional analgesics and co-analgesics by mouth according to the WHO analgesic ladder.[6] About 10% of patients have pain that is more difficult to manage and sometimes benefit from more complex interventions.[7]

Interventional pain management techniques can be highly effective. They may reduce the need for regular analgesia, with associated side-effects, for patients with malignant or non-malignant pain. In many countries improvements in palliative care and the scarcity of consultant anaesthetists with an interest in pain management have resulted in interventions being confined to patients with severe pain that is not adequately managed by simpler methods. This means that some patients are not offered potentially helpful interventions.

Patient selection

When reviewing the options for managing a patient's pain, there are situations that should trigger consideration of nerve blockade or neuromodulation.

- Pain persisting despite optimal oral analgesia.
- Effective oral analgesia resulting in intolerable side-effects.

- Rapid, effective analgesia required with limited time available for titration of oral analgesics or co-analgesics.
- Conditions that readily respond to nerve blocks (for example osteoarthritis of joints, ischaemic legs).

Individual techniques will be discussed in more detail in subsequent chapters, but in general the following should be considered:

Alternatives

It is important to manage pain with the simplest methods possible and to consider all available alternatives to an invasive technique. Simple nerve blocks may be easy to organize and are readily accepted by the patient (Fig. 1.1). They may be done at home or in the hospice with little or no aftercare. However, optimizing oral analgesia may be more acceptable, even when pain control is incomplete, if the alternative is a complex nerve block requiring hospital admission and extensive aftercare. The possibilities for

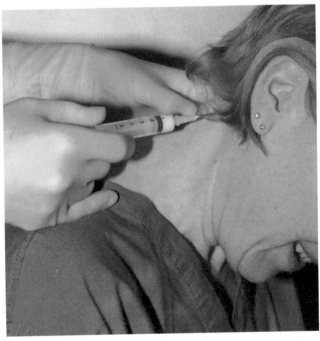

Fig. 1.1 Patient having a simple trigger point injection.

disease-modifying treatments should be fully explored. These may include surgery for fracture fixation or bowel obstruction, radiotherapy for bone metastases, chemotherapy for appropriate tumour types, anti-anginals or antibiotics.

Patient characteristics

The relative importance of patient characteristics will vary according to the type of procedure planned and the situation. Table 1.1 gives some examples of contra-indications to nerve-blocking techniques.

Multi-professional decision making

The multi-professional team is the foundation of good palliative care and will help patients through complex decision making about modes of treatment.

Table 1.1 Examples of contra-indications to nerve-blocking techniques

	Relative contra-indication	Absolute contra-indication*
Co-morbidity	Physical frailty Unable to sustain suitable position while nerve block is performed	Local or systemic sepsis, especially where an indwelling system is under consideration (see Chapter 5) Neutropenia/thrombocytopenia
Concomitant medication	Aspirin, clopidogrel, Low molecular weight heparin, Long-term steroids (risk of infection and delayed healing)	Warfarin, where stopping therapy for even a short period poses serious risk
Position of lesion	Risk of damage to healthy tissue such as intrathecal phenol, where bowel and/or bladder function are preserved	Impending spinal cord compression or raised intracranial pressure, where a spinal block is being considered
Mental state	Lack of capacity to make an informed choice	Unable to co-operate during the procedure and general anaesthesia not appropriate or possible

*For patients *in extremis*, there may be no absolute contra-indications when the benefits/burdens have been carefully weighed.

It is important to consider different perspectives regarding the patient and their pain and to explore other methods of pain management such as positioning of the patient, orthoses, and physiotherapy. The team must address psychological, social, and spiritual aspects of care that will have a bearing on the patient's physical pain. Using a physical technique to manage pain that has significant non-physical elements will result in disappointment. A careful assessment at the outset will avoid subjecting a patient to an invasive procedure with little chance of benefit.

Team issues

Where there are differing views about an intervention amongst team members these must be explored openly. Individuals weighing up the burdens and benefits of a course of action may come to different conclusions if the decision is finely balanced (Chapter 10). The success of any technique is never guaranteed. It is important that differences of opinion are aired before the procedure and a consensus is reached within the team as well as with the patient. If the procedure fails or complications occur, resulting recriminations can be highly destructive to the team and detrimental to patient care. However, when considering any intervention, team members must do this from a position of knowledge rather than prejudice. This requires support and explanation from the specialist that is often more time consuming than performing the block.

Communication

Good decision-making is dependent on good communication both within a team and between teams. When a nerve block or neuromodulation technique is being considered, a senior member of the palliative care service should make the referral to the pain team, discussing the patient's pain history, medical history, and other relevant information in detail. Where appropriate, the primary care team and other treating consultants should be involved. Following assessment by the pain service, detailed discussion about the options and preferred treatment plan is paramount, both with the patient and the referring teams. A patient's family and/or friends should be involved in any discussions at the patient's request. Patients must not be rushed into making decisions. It is important that they are given time to think about the options and to ask questions. Written information can be very helpful. Interventions may need to be performed urgently, but are rarely needed as an emergency and it should always be possible to allow a patient time to consider the alternatives.

Availability of a local pain management service

Options for treatment will depend on the availability of local expertise and ongoing support. Most palliative care patients with pain are frail and are not able to travel long distances for treatment or follow up. Where there is a request for 'long distance' pain control, investigation into what may be available locally is necessary before mentioning an interventional technique to a patient. It is not appropriate to raise expectations unless they can be met. Building relationships with local anaesthetic services and encouraging the development of a pain service may bear fruit in the medium term. However, pain specialists should not undertake procedures that they and the support staff are unfamiliar with, without appropriate supervision. Many complex interventions need regular clinical practice to maintain skills. There is no place for the occasional entrepreneur.

Availability of local facilities and support staff

In addition to local expertise, the availability of local facilities should be explored. Where a sophisticated pain service is available, access to anaesthesia, theatres, imaging, day case facilities or beds should not pose a problem— although getting interventions done urgently may be difficult. Where there is no such service, anaesthetic colleagues will have to consider the practicalities before accepting referrals. Undertaking complex interventions to provide complete pain relief in sub-optimal conditions (for example with inexperienced staff) may not be worth the risk. A simpler solution affording a lesser degree of analgesia may be preferred. Most nerve blocks and neuromodulation techniques are performed under local anaesthetic, and patient comfort and cooperation are of great importance (Fig. 1.2). Sedation or general anaesthesia may be needed in some cases and this should be discussed. The operator may sometimes give simple sedation him/herself, allowing verbal contact with the patient to be maintained throughout. This is only possible where there are trained staff available to monitor the patient during the procedure. When the procedure is to take place under general anaesthesia or heavy sedation, the patient should be told that the anaesthetic would be given by a separate anaesthetist who will assess their fitness. There is no situation that justifies a single operator-anaesthetist for this level of sedation/anaesthesia.

Patient choice

Patient choice is paramount to all decision making in palliative care and pain management. Where appropriate and at the patient's request, the family/carers

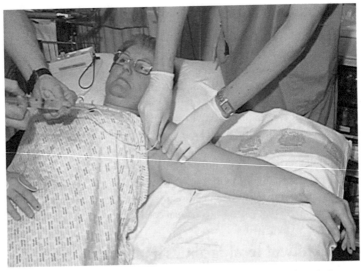

Fig. 1.2 Patient having a simple brachial plexus nerve block in hospital.

should be included in discussions. For a patient to make an informed choice, they must be fully apprised of all the options by an experienced professional who can discuss the details of any proposed procedure, the likely outcomes and possible adverse effects. The patient should be told the success and complication rate quoted in the literature, and within the actual unit. For some patients, good analgesia is their prime concern, even if there is a high risk of immobility after the procedure. Others would rather tolerate some pain in order to maintain their independence. Gaining true informed consent in these situations requires time and skilful communication. The person who is to perform the intervention must explain the nature of any proposed procedure in detail. Information should also be given about the nature of aftercare required and arrangements needed to continue care in the home.

Where to perform the intervention

Some very simple nerve blocks such as trigger point and joint injections may be performed in the patients home or in the hospice. Any procedure that involves placing a needle in the chest should only be done where there is the facility to rapidly site a chest drain. Any regional or spinal block, where there is the potential for toxic reactions or a total spinal anaesthetic, must be performed in hospital. Implantation of any long-term catheter or pump must be done in a clean-air operating theatre to minimize the risk of infection.

Aftercare

Decisions about aftercare must be made before any intervention is seriously considered. Some nerve blocks require little or no aftercare but patient safety must be balanced against convenience for more complex interventions. Immediate recovery from complex procedures is typically managed in the hospital post-anaesthesia care unit. Thereafter, most specialist palliative care services can then manage patients safely with advice from colleagues in anaesthesia. Patients who have been taking high dose opioids before any procedure, and for whom all sites of pain are likely to be substantially relieved, are at risk of opioid toxicity. The opioid dose should be significantly reduced (at least by 50%) immediately after the procedure. Careful nursing observation is paramount in the first hours to identify early signs of opioid toxicity and take appropriate action. Severe respiratory depression is a real risk. Conversely, patients whose pain does not respond as well as had been hoped may need extra analgesia.

Aftercare in the home may be more difficult immediately following an infusion technique—especially if drug doses are being titrated. Pharmacy colleagues may need to make up drug combinations for infusion in aseptic units and they must be involved in the early stages of planning the procedure to ensure that drugs are available promptly. When infusion doses are stabilized and home discharge is planned colleagues in primary care will be involved. They may be unfamiliar with such techniques. Where possible, district nurses and primary care doctors should be invited to the hospital to be trained in the ongoing management of the infusion. Information sheets including local guidelines and recommendations for practice are essential, and must include relevant contact numbers for advice both within and outside normal working hours. The patient should hold a copy of local guidelines in case any professional other than their usual primary care team needs such information. For patients who live at a distance from the centre where the procedure has been performed, discharge planning is even more complex and great care must be taken to ensure that appropriate backup is provided.

Summary

Simple nerve blocks can be done in the home or hospice following discussion within the multi-professional team and with the patient. Such procedures can afford excellent analgesia in selected circumstances.

When more complex blocks or infusion techniques are considered the following apply:

- Patients require careful evaluation
- Multi-professional team members are involved in decision making
- The patient must be carefully informed of the anticipated benefits and likelihood of complications
- Facilities and anaesthetic colleagues must be available and other relevant professionals should be involved from the early stages of planning
- The place of care after the intervention and immediate post-operative phase should be decided and arranged in advance

In such cases, performing the actual procedure is a small part of the total management of the patient's pain.

References

1. Vuorinen E (1993). Pain as an early symptom in cancer. *Clin J Pain* **9**:272–8.
2. Portenoy RK, Miransky J, Thaler HT, *et al.* (1992). Pain in ambulatory patients with lung or colon cancer. Prevalence, characteristics and effect. *Cancer* **70**:1616–24.
3. Donnelly S and Walsh D (1995). The symptoms of advanced cancer. *Semin Oncol* **22**(2 Suppl 3):67–72.
4. Addington-Hall J, Fakhoury W, and McCarthy M (1998). Specialist palliative care in non-malignant disease. *Palliat Med* **12**:417–27.
5. Addington-Hall J (1996). Dying from heart disease. *J Royal Coll Phys London* **30**(4):325–8.
6. WHO Expert Committee (1990). *Cancer pain relief in palliative care.* WHO technical report series 804, Geneva.
7. Cleeland CS, Gonin R, Hatfield AK, *et al.* (1994). Pain and its treatment in outpatients with metastatic cancer. *New Engl J Med* **330**:592–6.

2

Defining the problem

There are many factors that contribute to pain in patients who need palliative care. The incidence varies according to the underlying diagnosis and
stage of disease. For example, approximately 30–40% of patients with cancer
on active therapy report pain and this rises to 70–90% of patients with
advanced disease.[1] In one study 77% of patients with chronic lung disease
reported pain during the final year of life, with 56% saying that it was 'very
distressing'.[2] Similarly, a study of patients with end-stage heart failure
found that 32% suffered pain[3] and 65% of stroke patients experienced pain
in their last year of life.[4]

There are many causes of pain including:

The underlying disease
Malignant
- Visceral pain (for example liver capsule pain, bowel obstruction)
- Somatic pain (for example bone, wounds)
- Headache (for example raised intracranial pressure, meningeal disease)
- Neuropathic pain (for example intercostal nerve involvement, nerve
  entrapment with vertebral collapse, plexus invasion).

Non-malignant
- Ischaemia (for example angina, ischaemic limb pain)
- Musculo-skeletal pain (for example muscular dystrophies, arthritis,
  osteoporotic fractures (Fig. 2.1))
- Neuropathic pain (for example post-stroke pain, demyelination, AIDS-
  related neuropathy, diabetic neuropathy)
- Headache (for example migraine, tension headache).

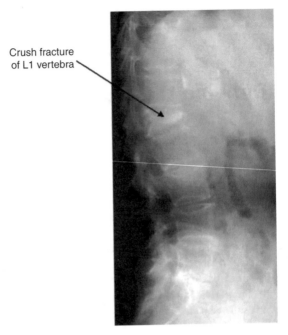

Crush fracture
of L1 vertebra

Fig. 2.1 Lateral X ray of a crush fracture of the L1 vertebra.

Treatments

Chemotherapy

- Mucositis
- Painful peripheral neuropathies
- Post lumbar puncture headache

Radiotherapy

- Strontium-89 induced tumour flare
- Radionecrosis

Surgery

- Wounds/drains
- Cannulae
- Phantom limb pain (Fig. 2.2)

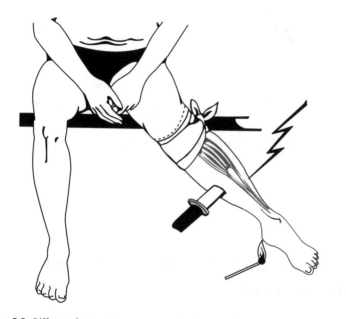

Fig. 2.2 Different facets of post-amputation limb problems, including phantom sensations, stump pain, neuroma pain, and phantom pain.

Drugs

- NSAIDs (dyspepsia, gastro-duodenal ulceration)
- Stimulant aperients (colic)

Investigations

Radiology

- Arteriograms
- Barium studies
- Positioning for CT or MRI scans

Endoscopy +/− stenting

- Ureteric
- Oesophageal

Biopsy

- Liver
- Skin

Debility

Infections

- Fungal (for example oral/oesophageal candida)
- Viral (for example herpes simplex, herpes zoster (Fig. 2.3))
- Bacterial (for example abscess, pneumonia, parotitis)

Reduced mobility and/or weight loss

- Joint pain and stiffness
- Myalgia
- Pressure sores
- Deep venous thrombosis

Co-existent disease/Pre-existing chronic pain

Musculoskeletal

- Osteoarthritis
- Frozen shoulder
- Muscle trigger spots

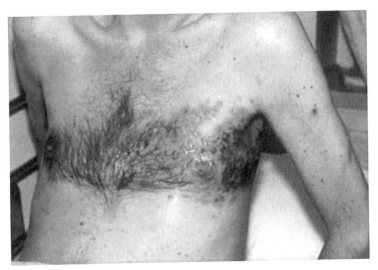

Fig. 2.3 Neuropathic pain: acute herpes zoster.

Vascular disease

- Ischaemic heart disease
- Peripheral vascular disease

Gastrointestinal disease

- Peptic ulceration
- Chronic pancreatis

Neurological

- Headache
- Post-stroke
- Neuropathies

Psychological/psychiatric problems

- Somataform pain disorder
- Anxiety
- Depression
- Addiction
- Illness behaviour and fear avoidance behaviour in patients with a long history of chronic pain (this group can be particularly difficult to assess)

Principles of pain management

Successful pain management depends on a logical, stepwise approach to treatment.

1 **Assess and treat each cause of pain**
Primary management involves establishing and reversing the cause of the pain where possible. For example, the appropriate use of antibiotics and/or drainage for infections/abscesses, internal or external fixation for fractures, spinal stabilization, aperients for the colic of constipation.

2 **Modify the disease process if the cause cannot be removed**
Where the cause of pain cannot be removed entirely, treatment should be directed at modifying the disease process if possible. Examples include using palliative radiotherapy and/or chemotherapy for malignant lesions, bisphosphonates for hypercalcaemia, bypass surgery for bowel obstruction, arterial stents or bypasses for ischaemic pain.

3 **Remove exacerbating factors**
If factors exacerbating the pain can be identified, they should be reviewed. For example, stimulant laxatives should be replaced with a more suitable alternative in the presence of bowel colic. For patients with dyspepsia, NSAIDs should be withdrawn or replaced with COX-2 inhibitors covered with a proton pump inhibitor.

4 **Explore the meaning of the pain for the patient**
In the context of palliative care with any underlying diagnosis, there is a spiritual element to many patients' pain. Worsening symptoms may be equated with the progression of disease and impending death. Suffering which challenges peoples world views may need to be addressed as patients struggle to make sense of issues of life, death, and meaning.

5 **Modify the social/physical environment where relevant**
Attention to a patient's physical environment is vital for the holistic management of pain. Comfort may be enhanced by the use of appropriate mattresses, orthotics, chairs, wheelchairs, stair lifts, and bathing facilities, for example. Working to maintain or introduce hobbies and interests in addition to enhancing the social environment may contribute to raising the pain tolerance and enhancing quality of life.

6 **Treat associated mood disorders**
Mood disorders are common in patients receiving palliative care. Depression and/or anxiety may worsen a patient's experience of his pain and should be diagnosed and treated with drug or non-drug measures as appropriate.

7 **Regular oral analgesics and co-analgesics, in accordance with the WHO analgesic ladder**[5, 6]
Most pains will be successfully managed as described in 1–7 above. For pain that persists or cannot be treated within acceptable limits of side-effects consider the following:

8 **Nerve block or neuromodulation technique**
Approximately 10% of pains in malignant disease are not relieved adequately by the above measures and require further evaluation and treatment.[7] The proportion of such pains in non-malignant disease is unknown. A nerve block or neuromodulation technique may be appropriate in some cases, and carries a high rate of success. For example, a coeliac plexus block has an 80% success rate.[8]

9 **Neurosurgery**
Cordotomy or other neurosurgical procedures may be necessary for a small number of patients with highly complex pain.

References

1. Portenoy R and Lesage P (1999). Management of cancer pain. *Pain* **353**: 1695–700.

2. Edmonds P, Karlson S, Khan S, *et al.* (2001). Comparison of palliative care needs of patients dying from chronic respiratory disease and lung cancer. *Palliat Med* **15**:287–95.

3. Anderson H, Ward C, Eardley A, *et al.* (2001). The concerns of patients under palliative care and a heart failure clinic are not being met. *Palliat Med* **15**:279–86.

4. Addington-Hall J, Lay M, Altman D, *et al.* (1995). Symptom control, communication with health professionals, and hospital care of stroke patients in the last year of life as reported by surviving family, friends and officials. *Stroke* **26**(12):2242–8.

5. Expert Working Group of the European Association for Palliative Care (1996). Morphine in cancer pain: modes of administration. *BMJ* **312**:823–6.

6. Expert Working Group of the European Association for Palliative Care (2001). Morphine and alternative opioids in cancer pain: The EAPC recommendations. *Br J Cancer* **84**(5):587–93.

7. Cleeland CS, Gonin R, Hatfield AK, *et al.* (1994). Pain and its treatment in patients with metastatic cancer. *New Engl J Med* **330**:592–6.

8. Eisenberg E, Carr DB, and Chalmers TC (1995). Neurolytic celiac plexus block for treatment of cancer pain: a meta-analysis. *Anesth Analg* **80**:290–5.

3

Assessment of pain

A detailed and thorough assessment is an essential prerequisite of successful pain management. For each site of pain, a careful history and physical examination is required. Some patients also need relevant investigations (for example bone scan, CT, or MRI scan). Treatment can then be tailored to the causes of pain. Accurate anatomical diagnosis is vital where a nerve blocking or neuromodulation technique is being considered as these are anatomically precise and will offer no analgesia if they miss the affected area. In contrast, oral analgesia will have a systemic effect.

Incidence

The incidence of pain in advanced cancer has been characterized to a much greater extent than pain in non-malignant advanced disease. Three quarters of patients with advanced cancer will experience pain, and these patients often have multiple sites and causes of pain. Approximately one-third have a single pain, one-third have two pains, and one-third have three or more pains;[1] 85% pains are due to the cancer itself, 15% are caused by general debility, a concurrent disorder or treatment.

Classification of pain

Nociceptive pain

Nociceptive pain is caused by actual or potential tissue damage. Classical descriptions of nociception involve cell damage that releases a range of local mediators that stimulate healthy Aδ and C nerve fibres to transmit pain signals to the spinal cord, along the spino-thalamic tract to the thalamus and higher centres. Nociceptive mechanisms are much more complex than this, many other pathways are involved in nociceptive processing. The nervous system is not hard-wired, but is plastic. It responds to afferent stimulation with neuronal and gene changes that occur rapidly in the periphery, spinal cord, and brain.[2] Nociceptive pain can be somatic or visceral.

Somatic pains are usually well localized, superficial, and often described as acute or sharp in nature.

Visceral pains are poorly localized, deep, and often described as dull or aching.

Neuropathic pain

Neuropathic pain is caused by dysfunction in nerve fibres, spinal cord, or brain (Fig. 3.1). Nerve compression or infiltration lead to altered sensation. Damage to peripheral nerves often leads to pain for example diabetic neuropathy or nerve ischaemia in peripheral vascular disease. When peripheral nerves are involved and this is sometimes referred to as deafferentationpain. Damage to autonomic nerves may cause sympathetically maintained pain. Damage to nerves within the central nervous system may cause central pain such as that seen following spinal cord compression, multiple sclerosis, or cerebrovascular events (see Chapter 4).

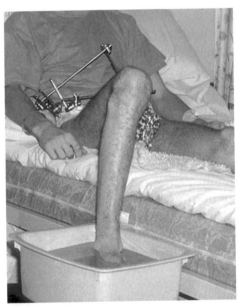

Fig. 3.1 Neuropathic leg pain in a man with traumatic sciatic nerve damage where the only ease was keeping his foot in warm water.

Neuropathic pain can also be *somatic* or *visceral*. Any pain in a region of reduced or altered sensation is neuropathic in origin. There are several concepts that may be helpful in the diagnosis of neuropathic pain:

Allodynia—pain evoked by a non-painful stimulus. It can be static such as with pressure or dynamic such as with stroking the area.

Hyperpathia—an increased reaction to a painful stimulus (often a repetitive stimulus) on the background of an increased pain threshold.

Hyperalgesia—a response of exaggerated severity following a painful stimulus.

Any of these findings are strongly suggestive of neuropathic pain.

Temporal variation of pain

Breakthrough pain is that which breaks through good pain control from background analgesia.[3] It can usually be successfully managed by increasing the dose of background drug treatment.

Incident pain occurs predictably given a particular stimulus. Examples include the movement-related pain of bone metastases or cough-related pain of pleurisy. Incident pains can be acute, severe, and disabling and are often short lived. They commonly do not respond well to the use of oral analgesics. Increasing the dose of background drugs causes sedation when the incident pain is not present. Nerve-blocking techniques can be particularly useful in the management of difficult pains such as incident pain.

Procedural pain is a particular type of incident pain that predictably occurs during a procedure, such as dressing changes.

Breakthrough, incident, and procedural pains can be either nociceptive or neuropathic in origin.

Table 3.1 gives examples of types of pain classified as nociceptive or neuropathic, somatic, or visceral.

Table 3.1 Examples of types of pain

	Nociceptive	Neuropathic
Somatic	Pressure sore Fracture Mucositis Arthritis	Post-herpetic neuralgia Brachial plexopathy Sciatica Diabetic neuropathy
Visceral	Peptic ulceration Large bowel colic Ischaemic bowel Myocardial infarction	Coeliac plexopathy from pancreatic cancer Para-aortic lymphadenopathy infiltrating visceral nerves

History

In taking a thorough pain history, each individual pain should be described in terms of:

- Site
- Radiation
- Intensity (at rest and on movement)
- Quality (looking for nociceptive and neuropathic features)
- Duration
- Temporal variation (relative to drug doses or activity)
- Previous therapies and their relative success
- Current therapies
- Precipitating factors
- Relieving factors
- Sleep
- Mood
- Activities of daily living
- Patient beliefs about the cause of pain.

The sites, radiations, and intensity of each pain can be drawn on a *pain diagram* as in Fig. 3.2, ideally by the patient himself. Not only can this assist in diagnosing the cause of each pain, but a good diagram can help when monitoring the success of any therapies.

Some patients also find it helpful to keep a *pain diary*. Grading the intensity of pain using a simple numerical rating scale (0–5) at rest, in relation to activity and to therapeutic interventions can help to clarify precipitating and relieving factors or the success of therapies. Some patients find the concept of numerical rating difficult and a verbal scale of none, mild, moderate, or severe may be preferable. Pain scales are available in many languages and may be downloaded and printed with English translations, from the British Pain Society.[4]

Plotting the sites and radiation of pain can also be useful in defining whether pain follows the distribution of particular dermatomes. A dermatomal distribution is pathognomic of neuropathic pain and determines which nerve roots are affected, thus helping to localize the lesion. However, it must be appreciated that many neuropathic pains do not have a dermatomal pattern.

Description of the quality of pain may point to a nociceptive or neuropathic cause.

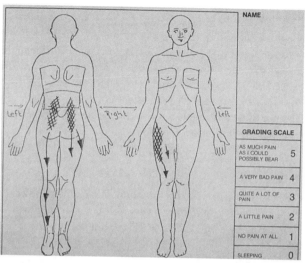

Fig. 3.2 A pain diagram where ### indicates the sites of pain and ↑ denotes the radiation of the pains.

Neuropathic pain is often described as 'pain in an area of altered sensation'. This implies sensory nerve damage and can be useful in the diagnosis of superficial neuropathic pains. Abnormal sensory qualities are a feature of neuropathic pain and the language used to describe the character of a pain may be useful in making the diagnosis. Descriptors such as pricking, tingling, numb, jumping, bursting, shooting, or stabbing are commonly used in addition to the symptoms described above. Autonomic changes may also be seen.[5]

Patients may demonstrate:

- Allodynia.

 Classical examples would be trigeminal neuralgia induced by cold air on the face or post thoracotomy pain that is excruciating when clothes rub gently against the affected area.

- Hyperpathia.

 An example of this would be pain from dressing a wound that may spread beyond the site of the wound or starts dull but winds up to an intense crescendo after repeated dressings.

- Hyperalgesia.

 An example of this would be severe pain induced by simple venepuncture in an affected area.

Examination

A thorough physical examination paying specific attention to possible causes of pain is essential for accurate diagnosis. This must include a full neurological assessment for the diagnosis of neuropathic pain. This also acts as a baseline if nerve blocks and neuromodulation are being considered. However, a history of altered sensation should be taken seriously even in the absence of demonstrable sensory changes, as sensory testing is not sufficiently sensitive to elucidate subtle signs.

Investigations

Where the cause of pain remains in doubt, or a detailed knowledge of a patient's pathology is required for a nerve-blocking technique to be considered, imaging by X ray, CT, or MRI scanning of the affected area is necessary.

Further reading

Twycross R (1997). *Symptom management in advanced cancer*. Radcliffe Medical Press, Oxford.

Ingham J and Portenoy R (1998). The measurement of pain and other symptoms. In: Doyle D, Hanks G, and MacDonald N (ed.), *Oxford textbook of palliative medicine*, 2nd edn., pp. 203–19. Oxford University Press, Oxford.

References

1. Grond S, Zech D, Diefenbach C, *et al.* (1996). Assessment of cancer pain: a prospective evaluation in 2266 cancer patients referred to a pain service. *Pain* **64**:107–14.
2. Aguggia M (2003). Neurophysiology of pain. *Neurol Sci.* **24**(Suppl 2):S57–60.
3. Portenoy RK and Hagen NA (1990). Breakthrough pain: characteristics and impact in patients with cancer pain. *Pain* **81**:129–34.
4. www.painsociety.org.
5. Bennett M (2001). The LANSS pain scale: the Leeds assessment of neuropathic symptoms and signs. *Pain* **92**:147–57.

4

Pain syndromes

Recognition of patterns of pain that occur in patients in the palliative phase of their disease can help the clinician to diagnose the most likely cause of pain, and decide on the most appropriate investigations and treatments. Patterns of pain in cancer have been well described[1–3] as cancer pain syndromes, but non-malignant pain is less well characterized. This chapter will highlight some of the pain syndromes in cancer and non-cancer palliative care and, where applicable, suggest suitable nerve blocks.

Cancer-related pain syndromes

These may be due to the cancer itself, diagnostic interventions, treatment for the cancer or its complications, or may be coincidental. It is helpful to divide pain syndromes into *acute* or *chronic* as this directs treatment options.

Acute pain syndromes
Acute pain associated with diagnostic procedures

Pain in this context, such as that associated with percutaneous biopsy or paracentesis, is usually very short-lived and well managed with oral analgesia, topical anaesthesia, or simple local anaesthetic infiltration. In some situations nitrous oxide:oxygen, as a 50:50 mixture, may be used as analgesia; it is effective if it is administered properly. Some pains may continue for a few hours or even a few days, such as post-lumbar puncture headache. These may be managed with a technique aimed specifically at the cause (for example epidural blood patch) or with analgesia that can be reduced in dose as the pain subsides. Nerve blocks are not normally of benefit in these situations.

Acute pain caused by therapeutic interventions

Pain caused by therapeutic interventions such as tumour embolization or nephrostomy insertion can usually be managed by appropriate local anaesthesia supplemented by oral or parenteral analgesia. The exception to this is *post-operative pain* that may extend over many days. Regional analgesia such as that afforded by a plexus or an epidural infusion can be highly effective in such circumstances. Care must be taken to continue to assess the patient's pain in a holistic manner and not to assume that the regional block will treat all sources of pain. Many patients will continue to require oral analgesics as prescribed before surgery to cover sources of pain outside the region of the block. If the patient develops a post-operative complication such as a wound infection, haematoma, or spinal cord compression, the block may mask this and so vigilance is needed. However, severe pain from such complications often breaks through the regional technique and should usually be apparent to observers. If the operation did not remove the original cause of pain then continuing analgesia will be necessary beyond the post-operative period.

Acute pain may also be associated with *chemotherapy*. Pain on administration suggests extravasation and must be treated immediately. Acute effects include diffuse bone pain, especially when treating leukaemias, and painful peripheral neuropathies after some agents (for example vinca alkaloids, cisplatin). *Hormone therapy*, especially for breast and prostate cancer, can cause an acute tumour flare that presents as acute pain. *Radiotherapy* can cause acute pain—for example from incident pain during the positioning of a patient, or from acute radiation proctocolitis. None of these types of acute pain would normally be managed with a nerve-blocking technique.

Acute infection

The cause of acute pain must always be investigated as appropriate to the patient's general condition. Acute infections may present with pain such as intra-abdominal abscess formation, pleurisy, mucositis, and herpes zoster. The most effective treatment is to clear the infection with appropriate antibacterials, antifungals, or antivirals. Surgical drainage of abscesses may be required. There is usually no place for nerve-blocking techniques in these circumstances.

Acute pain due to the cancer itself

Acute tumour-related pain can occur in a number of situations such as vertebral collapse, pathological fracture, intestinal obstruction, or haemorrhage into a tumour. Nerve blocks can sometimes be used as a temporary measure to treat vertebral collapse or pathological fractures whilst arranging more definitive treatment. If the initial insult cannot be treated (such as by pinning a pathological fracture) these acute pains may develop into chronic pain and the management will change.

Chronic pain syndromes

Chronic tumour-related pain syndromes

Nociceptive pain syndromes

Many tumour-related nociceptive pain syndromes respond well to nerve-blocking techniques if other, less complex, treatment modalities are not effective. Such syndromes include *bone, joint,* and *soft tissue* pain, *paraneoplastic* pain syndromes such as hypertrophic pulmonary osteoarthropathy and *visceral* pains due to neoplastic infiltration, such as liver capsule, pancreatic, or pelvic pain.

Bone pain is usually very well localized and, if the bone is superficial, there will be tenderness over the area (for example rib metastasis). Some bone metastases cause compression of related nerves, as that seen with base of skull metastases causing the orbital syndrome or middle cranial fossa syndrome.

Joint pains are well defined and precipitated by movement of the affected joint (for example hip metastasis or fracture).

Similarly, **soft tissue pain** is well localised, may be tender to touch if the area is superficial, or can be exacerbated by movement of the affected area, such as deep breathing or coughing with pleuritic pain. Some pain syndromes may be difficult to distinguish initially. The pain of rib metastasis, for example, can mimic pleuritic pain. Both will be well localized and worse on deep breathing or coughing. If the patient is asked to demonstrate the site of pain, the palm of the hand is usually used for pleuritic pain, whereas one finger is sufficient for rib pain. Careful examination will elicit the point tenderness of bone pain. As with all pain management, a detailed diagnosis is a vital prerequisite to choosing the best intervention for good pain control.

Visceral pain is caused by infiltration, compression, or obstruction of a viscus and usually presents little problem in diagnosis. Examples include:

- *Hepatic pain* from tumour or cholestasis, usually confined to the right upper quadrant, and worse on movement or deep inspiration. Pain may be referred to the ipsilateral shoulder tip.

- *Midline retroperitoneal syndrome* from carcinoma of the pancreas or retroperitoneal lymphadenpathy, causing back pain.

- *Chronic intestinal obstruction* causing constant background pain and colic.

- *Peritoneal carcinomatosis* causing constant abdominal or low back pain.

- *Malignant perineal pain* causing constant aching that is exacerbated by sitting or standing, and may be associated with tenesmus or bladder spasm.

- *Adrenal pain* that manifests as a unilateral flank pain, sometimes with associated generalized abdominal pain.

- *Ureteric obstruction* causing a constant dull flank pain, sometimes radiating to the ipsilateral inguinal region or genitalia.

Table 4.1 gives examples of nerve blocks to consider for nociceptive chronic pain syndromes.

Neuropathic pain syndromes

Neuropathic pain occurs with damage to peripheral or central nerves, or by aberrant somatosensory processing in the peripheral or central nervous systems.

It can involve:

- Individual peripheral nerves (**mononeuropathy**) such as femoral nerve compression by tumour
- Several nerves (**polyneuropathy**) such as tumour-related peripheral neuropathy (for example the peripheral neuropathy caused by cisplatin or vinca alkaloids)
- A nerve plexus (**plexopathy**) such as the cervical, brachial, lumbosacral, or sacral plexus, caused by tumour invasion, or plexitis following radiotherapy
- A nerve root (**radiculopathy**) affecting a single dermatome, usually caused by epidural tumour compression or invasion or leptomeningeal metastases
- The **spinal cord** as seen with epidural spinal cord compression
- **Central pain** that may include spinal cord pain.

Central pain is not well understood or researched and may be overlooked when trying to reach a diagnosis of the cause of pain. Many different types of lesion in the brain or spinal cord may cause pain. It may present with mild pain in a small area, but more commonly affects large areas of

Table 4.1 Blocks to consider for nociceptive chronic pain syndromes

Pain type	Site	Block to consider*
Bone pain	Rib	Intercostal block
	Vertebral collapse	Paravertebral block, epidural
	Hip fracture or metastasis	Lumbar psoas block
Soft tissue	Pleura	Intrapleural block
	Sarcoma of biceps	Brachial plexus block
Visceral	Liver capsule	Coeliac plexus block
	Pelvic pain	Superior hypogastric plexus block

*See Chapter 7 for further information including contra-indications.

Table 4.2 Blocks to consider for neuropathic chronic pain syndromes

Pain type	Site	Block to consider*
Mononeuropathy	Femoral nerve	Femoral nerve block
Polyneuropathy	Peripheral neuropathy	None effective
Plexopathy	Brachial plexus	Brachial plexus block
Radiculopathy	Thoracic root	Paravertebral block at level of lesion
Spinal cord	Lumbar region	Intrathecal infusion
Central pain	Brain	Deep brain stimulation

*See Chapter 7 for further information including contraindications.

the body causing severe distress. A diagnosis of central pain should not be made in the absence of pathology in the central nervous system.[4]

Table 4.2 gives examples of nerve blocks to consider for neuropathic chronic pain syndromes.

Chronic therapy-related pain syndromes

There are a variety of chronic pain syndromes that follow treatment for cancer and these may again be divided into nociceptive or neuropathic pains.

Nociceptive pain syndromes

Some of these syndromes may be amenable to nerve-blocking techniques. These include:

- **Bone** pain such as that from avascular necrosis of the hip following corticosteroid therapy or osteoradionecrosis; this may be helped by local injection.

- **Joint** pain such as that from a frozen shoulder following a long period of debility.

- **Soft tissue** pain such as that from gynaecomastia from hormone therapy for prostate cancer, painful lymphoedema following surgery or radiotherapy to axillary or inguinal lymph nodes.

- **Visceral** pain from chronic radiation enteritis or proctitis.

- **Chronic pelvic pain** due to radiotherapy.

- **Fungating tumours** may be very painful such as with breast or perineal malignancy, nerve blocks may sometimes be used to supplement local measures. Intrathecal phenol saddle block can be very helpful for perineal pain.

Neuropathic pain syndromes

Neuropathic pain syndromes can occur following chemotherapy, radiotherapy, or surgical treatments.

The most common chronic neuropathic pain following chemotherapy is the painful peripheral neuropathy associated with vinca alkaloids and cisplatin. This can also occur following treatment with paclitaxol. It presents in the classical 'glove and stocking' distribution, and is associated with hyporeflexia and autonomic changes. There is no good nerve-blocking technique that successfully manages this pain. The causative chemotherapeutic agents should be stopped at the first symptoms or signs of the development of a peripheral neuropathy. This prevents further damage, minimizing subsequent pain.

Radiotherapy can lead to fibrosis around nerve and nerve plexuses, causing cervical, brachial, or lumbosacral plexopathies, chronic radiation myelopathy, or radiation-induced peripheral nerve tumour. These are unusual, and can be minimized by careful attention to dosing and shielding areas where possible. Regional nerve blocks may be required in a few cases where pain is not adequately managed by other means.

It is not uncommon for surgery to result in chronic neuropathic pain, from injury to peripheral nerves or nerve plexuses. Syndromes include post-mastectomy pain that usually involves the area of the scar and ipsilateral arm, post-thoracotomy pain, and pain following radical neck dissection. In all cases patients must be evaluated carefully to exclude recurrent disease or infection, especially when pain begins some weeks after surgery and increases in intensity. All three syndromes may be managed with appropriate regional nerve blocks.

Phantom limb pain may occur following amputation and is more common in patients who have had significant and prolonged pain pre-operatively. Post-operative chemotherapy may be an additional risk factor. Phantom limb pain is perceived to come from the amputated limb as if it were still attached to the body. Pre- and post-operative nerve blockade are recommended for preventing phantom limb pains, however the evidence for this is poor. Phantom pains have also been described following other surgical procedures, such as breast pain post-mastectomy, bladder pain post-cystectomy, and anal pain following abdominoperineal resection of the rectum. If such pains develop months or years after surgery, they may herald recurrent disease.

Following any surgical incision, there may be neuroma formation within the scar or amputation stump. If this causes pain, it can be successfully treated by local injection with a depot steroid preparation and sometimes by small injections of a neurolytic (see Chapter 6).

Pain syndromes in non-malignant disease

Pain syndromes in non-malignant disease have been less well characterized. Nonetheless, there are certain syndromes that are important and relate either to general debility or to particular degenerative conditions. Many of these also occur in patients with cancer.

Muscle spasm

Painful muscle spasms occur in conditions where there is denervation of muscle, leading to uncontrolled muscle contraction. Such conditions include motor neurone disease (amyotrophic lateral sclerosis), multiple sclerosis, spinal cord compression or trauma, and Huntington's Chorea. Most patients gain adequate relief with oral muscle relaxants, but some may require other measures, such as local botulinum toxin injections or intrathecal baclofen (see Chapter 8).

Ischaemic pain

Arterial or venous insufficiency can result in ischaemic pain in any area (Fig. 4.1). This pain is characteristically at its worst when the requirement

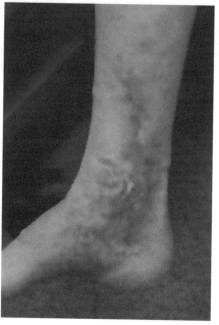

Fig. 4.1 Vascular leg ulcers.

for a good vascular supply is greatest. Mesenteric ischaemia therefore presents with abdominal pain after meals and refractory angina and leg ischaemia are worse during exercise. Autonomic neural blockade such as stellate ganglion blockade is effective for refractory angina and some ischaemic upper limb pains. Lumbar sympathetic blockade may improve the arterial supply to the legs affording good pain relief (see Chapter 7).

Neuromodulation using transcutaneous nerve stimulation or spinal cord stimulation may improve both blood supply and pain in ischaemia (see Chapter 9).

Musculoskeletal pains

Where there is muscle weakness, either from myopathy, neuropathy, or general debility, joint stability may be lost leading to subluxation or dislocation. This most commonly affects the shoulder but may occur at any joint. It is almost invariably painful. Positioning, orthoses, and physiotherapy are the mainstays of treatment but intra-articular injection may also be effective. Myofascial pain may occur where the patient has single or multiple muscle trigger spots that lead to local and/or referred pain. Local anaesthetic, steroid, or botulinum toxin injections may be used to treat muscle trigger spots (see Chapter 6).

Cutaneous pain

Chronic illness, poor nutrition, treatments such as steroid therapy and immobility all increase the risk of cutaneous pain caused by pressure necrosis. Although prevention aimed at the underlying risk factors is the most important aspect of care, some established pressure sores require analgesic therapy. In addition to the analgesic ladder and topical treatments, some painful sores may require a local or regional nerve block for debridement, dressing changes, or simply for general comfort.

Complex regional pain syndrome (CRPS)

CRPS is a term that covers several related conditions, including reflex sympathetic dystrophy, Sudeck's atrophy, and causalgia. It combines neuropathic pain with autonomic changes, trophic changes, inflammation, oedema, muscle spasm, and loss of function (Fig. 4.2). It is probably an array of similar syndromes, rather than a single entity that progresses stepwise through all stages in each case. There may be a genetic predisposition to CRPS. It is very debilitating and often associated with low mood. It may follow damage to:

- Peripheral tissues, such as fractures and dislocations, mastectomy and deep vein thrombosis

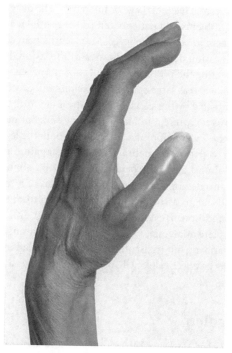

Fig. 4.2 Complex regional pain syndrome of hand where the skin is shiny and trophic.

- Peripheral nerves, such as brachial plexus lesions or post-herpetic neuralgia
- Central nervous system, such as cerebral infarction, tumour or spinal cord lesions
- Viscera, such as abdominal disease or myocardial infarction.

There is no single effective treatment for this syndrome but drug treatment combined with sympathetic blockade may be of benefit especially if it is combined with active physiotherapy (see Chapter 7) and spinal cord stimulation may be helpful (see Chapter 9).

Central pain

Central pain (a term that includes thalamic pain) may be caused by a lesion anywhere within the brain or spinal cord. In palliative care practice it can be found in conditions such as multiple sclerosis, Parkinson's disease, and following cerebral haemorrhage or infarction. The diagnosis of central pain can pose problems and patients can present with bizarre syndromes that may lead them to being disbelieved. Most central pain covers extensive areas, and its location depends on the area of the lesion. For example, a large lesion affecting the posterior limb of the internal capsule will cause hemibody pain, whereas large spinal cord lesions will cause bilateral pain in the area innervated by the affected segments of the cord. Central pain in multiple sclerosis can present in many different ways but most commonly causes pain in the lower half of the body, one or both the legs, arm and leg on one side, or as trigeminal neuralgia. As central pain is a sensory phenomenon it is almost always associated with sensory abnormalities with some patients also demonstrating motor loss or ataxia. It may be difficult to distinguish the signs associated with central pain from the underlying neurological condition. Treatment for central pain is difficult and rarely results in complete analgesia. Oral analgesics and co-analgesics are the mainstay of treatment, but transcutaneous nerve stimulation or deep brain stimulation may be effective (see Chapter 9). Neurosurgical techniques are sometimes required.

Further reading

Doyle D, Hanks G, and MacDonald N (ed.) (1998). *Oxford textbook of palliative medicine*, 2nd edn. Oxford University Press, Oxford.

Wall PD and Melzack R (ed.) (1999). *Textbook of pain*, 4th edn. Churchill Livingstone, Edinburgh.

References

1. Portenoy RK and Lesage P (1999). Management of cancer pain. *Lancet* **353**:1695–700.
2. Foley KM (1998). Cancer pain syndromes. In: Doyle D, Hanks G, and MacDonald N (ed.), *Oxford textbook of palliative medicine*, 2nd edn., pp. 322–31. Oxford University Press, Oxford.
3. Cherney N and Portenoy RK (1999). Cancer pain: principles of assessment and syndromes. In: Wall PD and Melzack R (ed.), *Textbook of pain*, 4th edn., pp. 1017–64. Churchill Livingstone, Edinburgh.
4. Boivie J (1999). Central pain. In: Wall PD and Melzack R (ed.), *Textbook of pain*, 4th edn., pp. 879–914. Churchill Livingstone, Edinburgh.

5

Choice of technique

Anaesthetists have used peripheral and regional nerve blocks or spinal drug delivery to manage patients with pain from cancer for many years. The techniques were originally developed because of a lack of other, better analgesic methods or, in some countries, as a response to limited resources. However, with the advent of more logical prescribing based on the World Health Organisation analgesic ladder and availability of a wider range of drugs and routes, these techniques are now used less frequently. The lack of suitably trained or interested pain management specialists may be another important factor in some cases. This is unfortunate because multi-modal therapy is more likely to succeed when pain is difficult to control.[1, 2]

- About 10–15% patients with cancer-related pain could be helped by nerve blocks. It is best to start with *simple peripheral nerve blocks* where possible, and progress to more *complex regional blocks* later. However, if pain is widespread or disease is progressing rapidly, it is unlikely that simple blocks will produce long-term benefit. It is sometimes better to perform a more definitive procedure, rather than put the patient through multiple different blocks.

- About 1–2% patients are suitable for *spinal drug delivery*.[3] Drugs can be given spinally either as single injections epidurally or intrathecally (Chapter 7), as a single dose of intrathecal neurolytic (Chapter 7) or by external or internal spinal infusions (Chapter 8). Single doses of epidural local anaesthetic and steroid may help with nerve root pain and pain from vertebral collapse. Intrathecal neurolysis may help perineal pain or tenesmus although it does carry risks and careful patient selection is essential. More complex pain problems are probably better served by spinal infusions.

- Pain in the head may be helped by *intracerebroventricular drug delivery*. This requires the help of an interested neurosurgeon.[4]

General principles of nerve blocks

There are certain general principles in the management of pain from cancer using nerve blocks.

- Patients should be referred early for consideration of interventions.

- The pain must be carefully assessed and investigated (using appropriate laboratory tests, radiology, and neurophysiology) to determine whether a nerve block is feasible and likely to help.

- Careful explanation to ensure the full understanding and consent of the patient is essential. Patients and carers must be given adequate time to think about interventions and ask questions.

- Those who are to be involved in the patient's care after the block must understand the nature of the procedure, what it can and cannot achieve, how to look after the patient and what the likely effects and side-effects will be.

- Nerve blocks must not cause functional defects. Neuro-destructive procedures must be selective of sensory or autonomic nerves and leave motor paths and sphincters intact.

Nerve blocks should not be regarded as a treatment given in isolation but must form part of an overall strategy for analgesia. Nerve blocks are often forgotten or left as a last resort, by which time the patient may be too ill to tolerate the technique or to come to a hospital for the more complex procedures. Careful selection of patients and timing of interventions is vital. Early discussion with colleagues in pain management services is essential. Anaesthetists should make themselves easily available for consultation about patients with difficult cancer pain and should offer prompt treatment. It is important that staff looking after patients with cancer can recognize pains that can be managed by nerve blocks and understand what each procedure entails so that appropriate and timely referrals can be made. Every intervention must be considered in terms of its possible benefits, what is needed of the patient, carers and staff, inconvenience, risks and recuperative time. The choice of techniques offered also depends on the skills and resources of the local pain management service. Referral to a tertiary centre for a single intervention, such as coeliac plexus block, may sometimes be appropriate if local expertise is not available. However, such referrals for techniques that need ongoing management, such as spinal drug delivery, may not be appropriate if local follow-up and after care is not available (see Chapter 1).

General indications for nerve blocks

- Somatic pain confined to a few dermatomes such as radicular limb pain
- Autonomic nerve involvement such as visceral pain, intractable angina
- Vascular pain.

General contraindications to nerve blocks

Absolute contraindications

- Patient refusal
- Local or systemic infection
- Non-correctable co-aggulopathy
- Lack of skilled pain management specialist
- Lack of support services in hospital, palliative care unit or community.

Relative contraindications

- Current chemotherapy and neutropenia (infusions or depot steroids)
- Neurological problems must be investigated and documented prior to any procedure. A nerve block may either mask or contribute to deterioration in neurological function.

Techniques, equipment, and environment

Nerve blocks may be performed as a single injection or may involve the placement of a catheter with an infusion of drugs from a pump.

Simple nerve blocks may be performed in a hospice setting. These include blocks such as trigger spot injections and intra-articular injection. These usually only require readily available equipment such as sterile supplies and short, bevelled nerve blocking needles (Fig. 5.1).

Complex techniques, with risks of adverse events, or those that require image intensification, must be performed in hospital. These include blocks such as brachial plexus and paravertebral blocks. The success rate of some more complex blocks may be improved by the use of a peripheral nerve stimulator and insulated needles. Electrical stimulation is then used to locate the needle tip close to nerves and nerve plexuses such as for brachial plexus block. Radiological imaging with or without the use of contrast medium is helpful

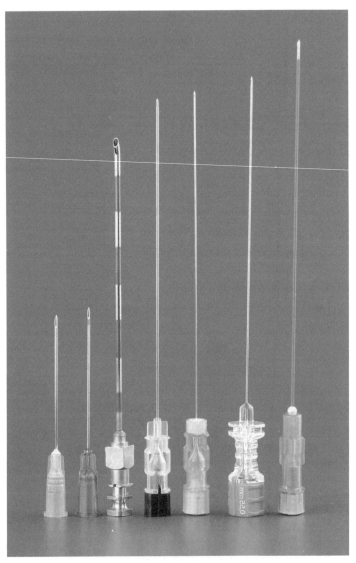

Fig. 5.1 Examples of needles used for nerve blocking. (From left to right) standard 21 G (gauge) green sharp bevelled injection needle, 22 G Huber side-holed needle used for intrathecal pump refills, 16 G Tuohy epidural needle marked in 1 cm graduations, 22 G short bevelled spinal needle, 24 G pencil point spinal needle, 22 G side-holed Sprotte spinal needle and radiofrequency lesioning probe.

for some blocks, such as psoas compartment block, and mandatory for others such as coeliac plexus block. Some operators use CT scanning for some of the more complex nerve blocks, however there is little evidence that it improves overall success rates and it does make the procedures more complex.

Radiofrequency lesions can be performed using fine probes that are placed on the target area, using fluoroscopy. A stimulating current is passed down the probe to check its position by inducing appropriate sensory effects and ensuring that motor nerves are not stimulated. Efficacy depends on accurate probe placement, as lesions are small. The patient needs to be awake and cooperative for this to be successful. Local anaesthetic is then injected down the probe prior to lesioning that is performed at 60–90°C for 60–120 seconds, depending on the area to be treated. Pulsed radiofrequency lesioning can also be used. In this situation the probe does not reach a high temperature but it is thought that the radiofrequency current itself has an analgesic effect. Re-innervation is almost inevitable after any radiofrequency technique but usually takes some months, after which the procedure can be repeated. This technique is not appropriate for peripheral nerves, as it can lead to increased pain after re-innervation and deafferentation pain.

Positioning the patient is part of the procedure. Most nerve blocks are much easier to perform if the patient can be positioned optimally and skilled assistance is available. There is no place for trying to do complex blocks with the patient poorly positioned in bed, with poor light, and an assistant who has never seen the procedure before. This renders the block more risky and likely to fail; it will prolong the intervention and thus increase the patient's distress and discomfort.

Choice of environment must be correct for the procedure. This may be a well-lit and equipped treatment room in a hospice, it may be a radiology suite or it may be a hospital operating theatre. The choice depends on the needs of the patient, the type of nerve block, and local circumstances.

Some blocks can be easily performed with the patient fully awake such as intercostal block. However, some patients require analgesia with anxiolytics or sedation so that they can be positioned and lie still for the procedure. A trained person must administer drugs and the patient must be adequately monitored throughout.

Some blocks, such as coeliac plexus block, require deep sedation or anaesthesia (Fig. 5.2). This requires the presence of an anaesthetist who is not the operator. It is not possible to perform complex nerve blocks whilst simultaneously monitoring the patient's conscious level and comfort.

Injections in the root of the neck or chest wall carry the risk of tension pneumothorax and must only be performed where it is possible easily and rapidly to insert a chest drain.

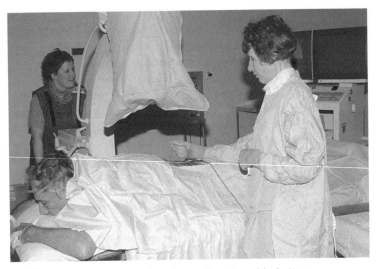

Fig. 5.2 Patient in theatre undergoing coeliac plexus block. Note prone position, full anaesthetic monitoring, venous access, surgical drapes, fluoroscopy, and full asepsis required.

A serious complication of injection near the spine (such as during an epidural, stellate, or paravertebral block) is accidental subarachnoid administration of a large volume of local anaesthetic – a 'total spinal'. This produces brain stem paralysis with devastating cardio-respiratory collapse within minutes. Resuscitation requires tracheal intubation, ventilation, and circulatory support with fluids and vasopressors.

Only those competent to manage all the possible adverse effects in an appropriately staffed and equipped environment should perform complex nerve blocks and use potentially toxic doses of drugs.

Drugs used for nerve blocks

A clear understanding of the pharmacology of the drugs involved is vital so that the appropriate agents can be chosen for the task and side-effects anticipated and managed.

Single injections usually use local anaesthetic; long acting agents such as bupivacaine, levobupivacaine, and ropivacaine are probably the most appropriate. This may be combined with injection of steroid whose local effects depend on potency, solubility, and dose. Hydrocortisone is a weak anti-inflammatory agent that is absorbed quickly and has an effect that often only lasts a few days. The synthetic steroids such as triamcinolone hexacetonide, triamcinolone acetonide, or methylprednisolone acetate are about five times more potent and less soluble; their effect can last weeks or months. Systemic absorption after injection may be sufficient to reduce inflammation in areas that have not been injected. It is possible that high or repeated doses may suppress the hypothalamic-pituitary-adrenal axis. Injections should probably not be repeated more often than every 8–12 weeks. There is controversy about the use of depot steroids epidurally, but there is no animal or clinical evidence that they are neurotoxic in the doses administered. Opioids may be used peripherally and there is some evidence that opioids are effective analgesics when they are injected into joints. Botulinum toxin may be used to treat painful muscle trigger spots and spasticity.[5] Water-soluble non-ionic contrast may be used during some injections to localize the needle. It is important to check if a patient has a history of problems after contrast administration.

Chemical neurolysis has been practiced for about 140 years. Phenol, ethyl alcohol, and glycerol are the most commonly used agents.

Phenol neurolytic mixture is a combination of carbolic acid, phenic acid, phenylic acid, phenyl hydroxide, hydroxybenzene, and oxybenzene. It is prepared in water or in glycerine. Phenol has a local anaesthetic effect and so is not painful to inject. It may be mixed with contrast—but this dilutes its effect. It is highly soluble in glycerine and diffuses from it slowly. This is an advantage when it is given intrathecally as it allows limited spread and localized fixation to neural tissues. It is also hyperbaric and so careful positioning of the patient with the affected nerve down can control its spread in spinal fluid. When phenol in water is used its effect is much more neurolytic such as for chemical sympathectomy. A concentration of at least 7–8% is needed for neurolysis. It may take 24–48 hours after injection for the full effect to be manifest. Larger systemic doses of phenol (>8.5 g) are toxic leading to seizures and cardiovascular and central nervous system depression. Usual clinical doses of less than 1000 mg are unlikely to cause side-effects.

Ethyl alcohol is available as absolute alcohol with >95% concentration. Perineural alcohol injection is very painful; it is not used peripherally. It is hypobaric relative to spinal fluid and placing the patient with the affected side up can control its spread. It spreads readily in spinal fluid and so is not now commonly used intrathecally. The volume of neurolytic needed for coeliac plexus block is too great to allow the use of phenol so alcohol is the agent of choice. It is less toxic and 90–98% is completely metabolized.

Glycerol is used for neurolysis of the trigeminal ganglion. It is considered a mild neurolytic; however, like all of these agents there is potential for adverse effects on motor function and sphincters.

Infusions are usually local anaesthetic—occasionally with adjuvants such as opioids (Chapter 8) or clonidine (Chapter 8). The most commonly used local anaesthetics are lignocaine, bupivacaine, and ropivacaine. Lignocaine has the most rapid onset, but shortest duration of action. Bupivacaine is long lasting but has greater cardiovascular toxicity than levobupivacaine or ropivacaine. The former must not be used if there is a risk of absorption of a large dose. The effect of local anaesthetics is influenced by many factors the most important of which is the total dose used. As the dose increases, the onset of action is faster and the duration of effect longer. The proximity of injection to nervous tissue, nerve fibre diameter, and vascularity of the area all affect the onset and duration of block. It is important to calculate the toxic dose of local anaesthetic allowed in each patient and to stay well within the dose limit. Systemic toxicity of local anaesthetics is a continuum that depends on blood, myocardial, and brain drug concentrations. Systemic toxicity commonly occurs due to inadvertent intravascular injection or administration of too high a dose. The main toxic effects are central nervous and cardiovascular. The cardiovascular system is 4–7 times more resistant to these effects so seizures will usually occur before cardiovascular collapse. However, the myocardial toxicity of bupivacaine is long lasting and difficult to reverse.

General complications of nerve blocks

- Vasovagal collapse
- Local pain after injection; this is usually mild and treated with simple analgesics or anti-inflammatory drugs
- Allergy to injected drugs
- Toxicity of injected drugs
- Nerve or spinal cord damage from direct needle trauma
- Side-effects from unopposed actions of systemic drugs such as opioids. This may result in opioid toxicity from a patient's usual dose of systemic opioids when their pain is relieved by a nerve block.

Aftercare

This is as important as the procedure. Patients must be observed carefully after nerve blocks especially if they have received sedation or anaesthesia. If the nerve block takes effect quickly then patients may become sedated or develop respiratory depression due to the unopposed effects of their systemic drugs. It is important to anticipate this and adjust their medication appropriately. Patients require monitoring for some hours after a block; the duration and intensity of observations depend on the procedure performed and the patient's general condition. There should be local recommendations for monitoring after different procedures, to include oxygen saturation, respiratory rate, pulse, and blood pressure as a minimum.

Further reading

Patt RB (1998). The current status of anesthetic approaches to cancer pain management. In: Payne R, Patt RB, and Stratton-Hill C (ed.), *Assessment and treatment of cancer pain*, pp. 195–212. IASP Press, Seattle.

References

1. Miguel R (2000). Interventional treatment of cancer pain: the fourth step in the World Health Organization analgesic ladder? *Cancer Control* **7**:149–56.
2. Lordon SP (2002). Interventional approach to cancer pain. *Curr Pain Headache Rep* **6**:202–6.
3. Krames E (1999). Practical issues when using neuraxial infusion. *Oncology* **13**(Suppl 2):37–44.
4. Ballantyne JC, Carr DB, Berkley CS, *et al.* (1996). Comparative efficacy of epidural, subarachnoid, and intracerebroventricular opioids in patients with pain due to cancer. *Reg Anesth* **21**:542–56.
5. Royal MA (2003). Botulinum toxins in pain management. *Phys Med Rehabil Clin N Am* **14**:805–20.

6

Simple peripheral nerve blocks and injections

Some simple nerve blocks and injections can provide excellent symptomatic relief with minimal discomfort and risk for the patient. Many of these techniques can be learned easily and may be undertaken by a variety of clinicians. Some more complex blocks, such as facet and dorsal root injections, need more experience. Most simple blocks can be performed with quite basic equipment, attention to asepsis, and in a clean environment. However, some blocks are more successful if fluoroscopy is used, with radio-opaque contrast where appropriate. Most simple techniques use local anaesthetic usually with depot steroid (Chapter 5). Sometimes repeated blocks with local anaesthetic alone produces analgesia far in excess of the duration of the local block. Botulinum toxin can be used for some muscle 'trigger point' injections and for spasticity, and may produce about 3–4 months benefit. Radiofrequency lesioning can be used to produce a more prolonged effect in some cases, such as with facet joint blocks. Minimal aftercare is usually needed following simple nerve blocks.

General indications

- Pain from cancer such as painful bony metastasis
- Pain from cancer treatment such as scar or stump pain
- Pain due to general debility such as muscle pain
- Coincidental pain such as nerve entrapments, degenerative joints, chronic spinal pain
- Incident pain, but blocks may require repeating
- Whilst awaiting a more definitive analgesic therapy such as radiotherapy or a more interventional nerve block.

Metastasis injection

Painful metastases may be injected with a combination of local anaesthetic and depot steroid usually using fluoroscopy to aid needle placement (Fig. 6.1). A combination of local anaesthetic and depot steroid is usually used. It is important not to exceed the maximum dose of local anaesthetic as injection into a vascular metastasis may lead to rapid systemic absorption. The effect of the local anaesthetic wears off within hours; the duration depends on the drug used, the site of injection, and the vascularity of the lesion injected. The steroid may then take some days to be effective. Opioids can be injected into peripheral sites; they have an anti-inflammatory and analgesic action. There can be an increase in pain once the local anaesthetic has worn off and this should be pre-empted by giving oral analgesics. If the injection is helpful it can be repeated every 6–8 weeks, taking into account the maximum recommended dose of the steroid.

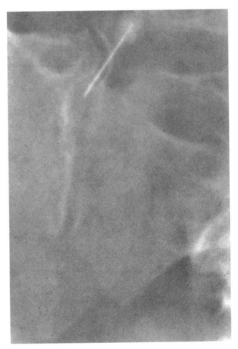

Fig. 6.1 Injection to painful metastasis near sacroiliac joint under fluoroscopy.

Scar or stump injection

Patients may have pain due to nerve entrapments in scar tissue or amputation stumps. Injections may not be of benefit in patients with widespread scar or stump pain where accurate localization of 'trigger points' is not possible. If there are definite localized areas of tenderness in the area, with or without a positive Tinnell's sign, then local infiltration may be worthwhile. This can be very painful. It may be useful to apply a topical preparation such as EMLA (Eutectic Mixture of Local Anaesthetics) cream for two hours prior to the procedure. Care should be taken to use the smallest needle possible and inject gently and slowly (Fig. 6.2). Local anaesthetic with or without depot steroid may be used. It may be preferable to perform serial simple local anaesthetic injections.

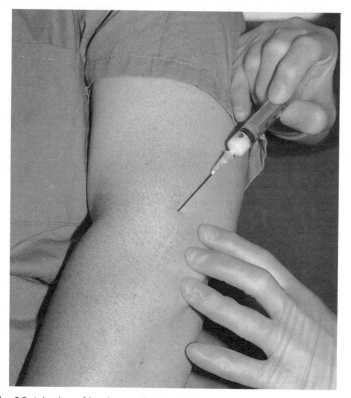

Fig. 6.2 Injection of local anaesthetic and depot steroid into a painful scar on the elbow.

Myofascial 'trigger point' injection

Myofascial pain may occur as a result of trauma, underlying problems (such as back pain, headache, or visceral pain), or due to general debility and poor posture. Patients may develop one or many painful muscle 'trigger points' as part of a myofascial pain syndrome.[1, 2] These are hyperirritable loci within a band of skeletal muscle or its associated fascia that are painful on palpation. Pressure over the area reproduces the pain and often results in pain that can radiate quite widely. Sometimes a taught band of muscle can be felt. Palpation may result in the muscle visibly contracting, and patients may also exhibit a jump sign and a twitch response. There is increased electromyographic activity in trigger pints that is made more prominent by a psychological stressor.[3] There can be associated autonomic dysfunction such as localized changes in skin temperature and sweating. Careful clinical examination and experience is needed to localize the 'trigger point' accurately. There is improved inter-observer reliability in finding trigger points following a training period.[4] Pressure sensitive devices can also aid identification of trigger points.[5]

Each painful 'trigger point' can be injected with 2–3 ml of a long-acting local anaesthetic such as bupivacaine or ropivacaine, using a fine needle and gentle, slow injection (Fig. 6.3). Depot steroid may be used on the first occasion, but a repeated steroid injection into muscle 'trigger points' over a protracted period is not recommended, as this may lead to fibrosis. Sometimes repeated, accurate injections of local anaesthetic are helpful. If this produces an effective, but short-term response, then the botulinum toxin can be used. This lasts about 3–4 months and can be repeated.[6–8] Minimal aftercare is needed following 'trigger point' injection. Pain may increase for a few days after the injection and patients should take simple analgesics as necessary. Injections should always be combined with regular exercises aimed at stretching the affected muscles. Supervision by a physiotherapist is therefore very useful for these patients.

Myofacial pain syndrome should be distinguished from fibromyalgia.[9] This syndrome involves a large number of painful 'trigger spots' and sleep disturbance with associated behavioural changes. Fibromyalgia is not helped by injections and patients are often made worse by such invasive treatments.

Peripheral nerve blocks

Sometimes simple superficial peripheral nerve blocks can be useful. These require a sound knowledge of the local anatomy, and some experience. Local anaesthetic with or without depot steroids can be used.

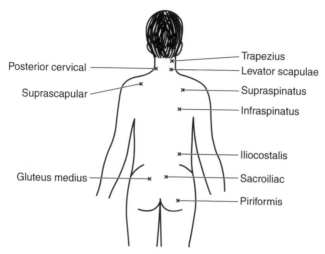

Fig. 6.3 Some common sites for injection of myofascial trigger points.

Pulsed radiofrequency lesioning has been suggested though there is no good evidence base for this. Standard radiofrequency lesioning and injection of neurolytic should not be used on peripheral nerves, as these are likely to cause deafferentation pain.

Examples of techniques include:

- *Greater occipital nerve block* can be used unilaterally or bilaterally for posterior head pain that often radiates anteriorly to the eye. Pain may be due to degenerative problems or local nerve entrapment. The block involves injection of 3–5 ml local anaesthetic with or without steroid between the mastoid process and greater occipital protuberance into the muscle layer where the nerve lies.

- *Suprascapular nerve block* can be very useful in patients with shoulder pain either alone or as an adjunct to intra-articular shoulder injection.[10] A catheter technique has been described to allow repeated doses of local anaesthetic.[11] The block is performed by using a small needle to inject 5 ml local anaesthetic and steroid over the midpoint of the upper border of the scapula. The nerve lies in a groove, however deep injection should be avoided because of the risk of damaging the nerve and of producing a pneumothorax.

- *Upper limb blocks* such as to the ulnar, radial, or median nerve can be used to treat nerve entrapments or provide analgesia for procedures.

These blocks are very simple to perform. Patients may experience transient motor weakness for the duration of the local anaesthetic and they must be warned to protect the limb during this time.

- *Ilioinguinal* and *iliohypogastric* nerves may be blocked in the groin to treat nerve entrapments or pain in surgical scars.

- *Femoral nerve block* may be useful in patients with pain in the hip or to reduce muscle spasm in patients with femoral fractures or metastases (Fig. 6.4). This approach can be useful for incident pain or as a temporary measure whilst more definitive treatment is organized. The femoral nerve is blocked by injecting lateral to the femoral artery in the groin. A volume of 10 ml local anaesthetic is usually sufficient. Care must be taken to avoid intravascular injection. A catheter may be placed in the femoral canal to allow repeated injection or infusion of local anaesthetic. Catheters cannot be used long-term in this area because of difficulty with fixation and infection risk. To provide total analgesia for the hip it is necessary to block the obturator, sciatic, and lateral cutaneous nerve of the thigh. This can be achieved in some patients by a '3 in 1 block' where a larger volume of 20–25 ml local anaesthetic is injected around the femoral nerve with distal pressure to force the solution proximally. Care must be taken to avoid toxic doses of local anaesthetic. Hip and leg pain may be better addressed by a psoas compartment block for unilateral pain (Chapter 7) or a spinal technique (Chapter 8) for bilateral pain.

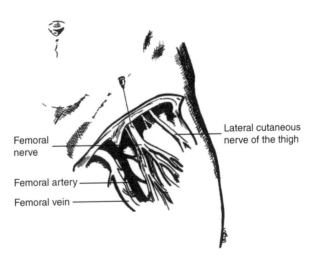

Fig. 6.4 Femoral nerve block. The injection is performed lateral to the vein and artery in the groin.

- *Lower limb blocks* such as to the common peroneal and tibial nerves may be used to treat nerve entrapments or provide analgesia for procedures. These blocks are very simple to perform. Patients may experience transient motor weakness for the duration of the local anaesthetic, and they must be warned to protect the limb during this time.

Joint injections

Intra-articular injections can be used for a variety of joint pains such as shoulder, hip, or knee[12] (Fig. 6.5). These are simple to perform, but better results are often obtained when injection is guided by the use of fluoroscopy and radio-opaque contrast. Local anaesthetic and depot

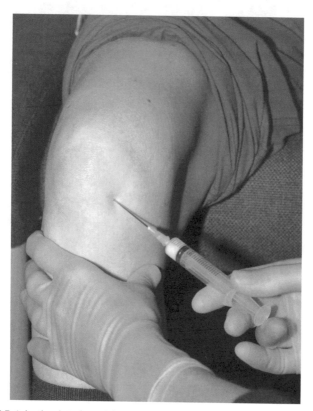

Fig. 6.5 Injection into knee joint.

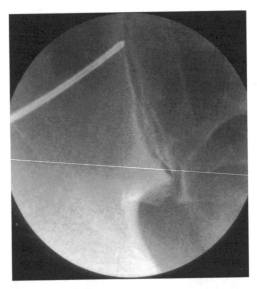

Fig. 6.6 Sacroiliac joint injection.

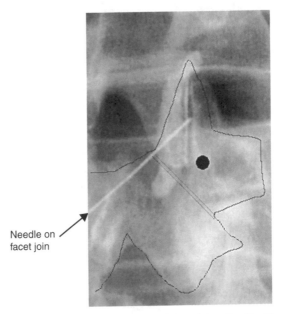

Needle on
facet join

Fig. 6.7 Oblique view of injection of a spinal facet joint. The 'Scottie dog' outline allows visualization of the joint. Injection is around the joint above the eye of the dog.

steroid injection are commonly used; the dose and volume are dependent on the size of the joint and severity of pain. Opioids can be injected into inflamed joints but the evidence base for this practice is small. Patients should be warned that pain and stiffness might increase after injection and the analgesic effect may be delayed. Painful sacro-iliac joints can be injected with local anaesthetic and steroid using fluoroscopy (Fig. 6.6). If only temporary benefit is achieved then radio frequency lesioning can be used.

Spinal injections

A variety of injections to the spine are possible for patients with degenerative back problems; these blocks are well described in standard textbooks and include facet joint (Fig. 6.7) and dorsal root blocks (Fig. 6.8). The blocks can be performed at any level in the spine. These injections require fluoroscopy, and should only be undertaken by experienced practitioners. Initial injection of local anaesthetic can be followed by pulsed or standard radiofrequency lesioning as appropriate.

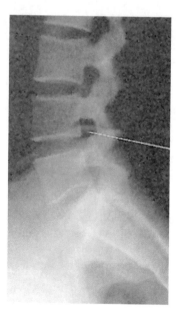

Fig. 6.8 Lateral X ray of dorsal root ganglion injection; the needle is placed in the intervertebral foramen.

Further reading

Baldry PE (1993). *Acupuncture, trigger points and musculo-skeletal pain*, 2nd edn. Churchill Livingstone, Edinburgh.

Brown DL (1999). *Atlas of regional anesthesia*, 2nd edn. W B Saunders Company, Philadelphia, PA.

Hahn MB, McQuillan PM, and Sheplock GJ (1996). *Regional anaesthesia: an atlas of anatomy and techniques*. Mosby, St Louis, MO.

Raj PP, Lou L, Erdine S, *et al.* (2003). *Radiographic imaging for regional anaesthesia and pain management*. Churchill Livingstone, Edinburgh.

References

1. Borg-Stein J and Simons DG (2002). Focused review: myofascial pain. *Arch Phys Med Rehabil* **83**(3 Suppl 1):S40–9.

2. Alvarez DJ and Rockwell PG (2002). Trigger points: diagnosis and management. *Am Fam Physician* **65**:653–60.

3. McNulty WH, Gevirtz RN, Hubbard DR, *et al.* (1994). Needle electromyographic evaluation of trigger point response to a psychological stressor. *Psychophysiology* **31**:313–16.

4. Gerwin RD, Shannon S, Hong CZ, *et al.* (1997). Inter-rater reliability in myofascial trigger point examination. *Pain* **69**:65–73.

5. Delaney GA and McKee AC (1993). Inter and intra-rater reliability of the pressure threshold meter in measurement of myofascial trigger point sensitivity. *Am J Phys Med Rehabil* **72**:136–9.

6. Royal MA (2003) Botulinum toxins in pain management. *Phys Med Rehabil Clin N Am* **14**:805–20.

7. Lang AM (2003). Botulinum toxin type A therapy in chronic pain disorders. *Arch Phys Med Rehabil* **84**(3 Suppl 1):S69–73.

8. Argoff CE (2002). A focused review on the use of botulinum toxins for neuropathic pain. *Clin J Pain* **18**(6 Suppl):S177–81.

9. Cymet TC (2003). A practical approach to fibromyalgia. *J Natl Med Assoc* **95**:278–85.

10. Mercadante S, Sapio M, and Villari P (1995). Suprascapular nerve block by catheter for breakthrough shoulder cancer pain. *Reg Anesth* **20**:343–6.

11. Emery P, Bowman S, Wedderburn L, *et al.* (1989). Suprascapular nerve block for chronic shoulder pain in rheumatoid arthritis. *BMJ* **299**:1079–80.

12. Anon (1995). Articular and periarticular corticosteroid injections. *Drug Ther Bull* **33**:67–70.

7

Regional nerve blocks

There is a variety of regional nerve blocks that allow interruption of individual nerves, plexuses, or ganglia that can be used for managing cancer pain. These are usually more technically demanding than the peripheral nerve blocks and injections and often have more serious potential complications. Anaesthetists with training in pain management most often perform these procedures though sometimes other specialists such as radiologists, surgeons, and rheumatologists undertake them. It is important that the operator has adequate training in the techniques and is proficient at resuscitation. They should perform the procedures often enough to maintain skills. Venous access should be established and transcutaneous oxygen saturation, ECG, and blood pressure monitoring should be instituted before and during any regional block. Regional nerve blocks must only be undertaken in an environment that provides adequate facilities for skilled assistance, sterility, monitoring, equipment, appropriate imaging, resuscitation, and aftercare.

- A single prognostic block using local anaesthetic can be used to predict the efficacy of a catheter technique or neurolytic block. These must be interpreted with caution as they can provide a powerful placebo effect and false positive results are common. If large doses of local anaesthetic are used, systemic absorption may produce analgesia from central effects that may be confusing. However, used carefully, prognostic blocks can be a way to assess whether an intervention can be performed easily and to demonstrate its effectiveness to patients and their carers.

- *A single therapeutic block* using local anaesthetic and depot steroid can be used. This can be repeated every few months if it produces benefit. However, care should be taken when using depot steroids not to exceed the maximum recommended dose. If there is disease progression and worsening pain then single 'one-off' nerve blocks become less likely to be of help.

- *Neurolytic blocks* may give months of relief. These may be repeated if necessary but may become more difficult if there is fibrosis after the first procedure. They are only used in patients with short life expectancies or where other simpler techniques have failed.

- *Infusion techniques* using catheters are needed in some situations, often for the management of complex or progressive pains. In patients with breakthrough or incident pain, catheter techniques may be used to give boluses before stimuli that provoke pain. Sometimes temporary catheters can be used to get pain control whilst waiting for a more definitive procedure such as radiotherapy or surgery.
- *Radiofrequency lesioning* (Chapter 5) can be used to destroy neural tissue in some circumstances such as trigeminal or sympathetic blockade.

Trigeminal ganglion block

Destruction of the trigeminal ganglion was reported nearly 100 years ago as a treatment for trigeminal neuralgia. This technique is still used in some patients who are not fit to undergo surgical decompression of the nerve. It also still has a place in the management of facial pain due to head and neck cancers.[1, 2] It involves lesioning near the base of the skull. A good knowledge of anatomy is mandatory and the block must be performed under fluoroscopy. The area is very vascular and may be distorted by tumour spread.

Specific indications

- Unilateral facial pain such as perineural tumour invasion
- Trigeminal neuralgia
- Facial pain from multiple sclerosis.

Specific contraindications

- Patients with cardiac conduction problems such as heart block may develop dangerous arrhythmias during trigeminal ganglionolyis
- Tumour invasion of the skull base that distorts the anatomy to an extent that renders the block too hazardous
- Patients who cannot lie still and co-operate fully with the procedure.

Anatomy

The 12 cranial nerves and the upper four cervical nerves supply the structures of the head and neck. Much of the innervation subserves special senses. The nerves that serve somatic functions contain only sensory or motor fibres. Thus, sensory blockade can be achieved without muscle paralysis. The trigeminal nerve is the largest cranial nerve and the most important target. It supplies sensation to the face, most of the scalp, the cornea, nasal cavity, mouth, and teeth. It also controls the muscles of mastication. The trigeminal ganglion lies in the foramen ovale in the middle cranial fossa, near the apex of the petrous temporal bone (Fig. 7.1). The ganglion is bounded medially by the cavernous sinus, superiorly by the inferior surface of the temporal lobe and posteriorly by the brain stem. The ganglion's posterior two-thirds is enveloped in a reflection of dura; intrathecal puncture is therefore possible when needling this area. The sensory root leaves the ganglion and divides into three divisions from dorsal to ventral: the ophthalmic, maxillary, and mandibular nerves that supply cutaneous sensation to the head. The smaller motor nerve root lies inferior to the ganglion and joins the mandibular division.

Techniques

Radiofrequency or neurolytic lesions can be performed with the patient supine, awake, and able to co-operate, so only light sedation should be given. Fluoroscopy in two planes is used to locate the foramen ovale on the affected side (Fig. 7.2). After local anaesthetic infiltration, a needle or

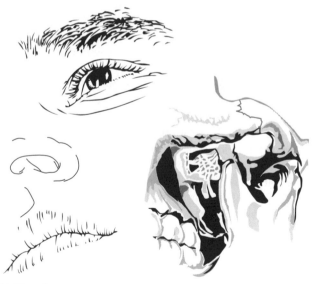

Fig. 7.1 The trigeminal ganglion.

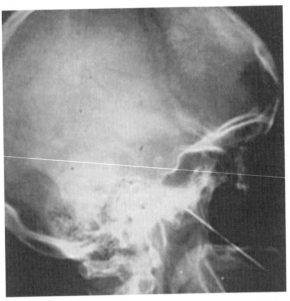

Fig. 7.2 Lateral view of trigeminal ganglion block with the needle in the foramen ovale.

radiofrequency probe is inserted 2–3 cm lateral to the angle of the mouth and medial to the masseter. It is directed to lie 3 cm anterior to the external auditory meatus on the lateral fluoroscopic view. In practice this usually means that the needle is aimed towards the ipsilateral pupil. The mandibular division of the nerve lies on the lateral side of the foramen, and the ophthalmic and maxillary divisions are more medial. Once the needle is in position, a small volume of radio-opaque contrast is used to verify its position, and ensure that it is not intrathecal. A diagnostic block can be performed with 1 ml local anaesthetic. This also helps to ensure that the needle is not intrathecal, when headache, fourth or sixth cranial nerve palsy, or pupil changes may be seen. If the needle position is satisfactory, up to 1 ml of neurolytic may be given in 0.1 ml aliquots. However, neurolytic is not commonly used now and radiofrequency lesioning is probably preferable as this has fewer risks.

Injection of glycerol is a simpler technique and it is a gentler neurolytic. It may be applicable when patients cannot tolerate radiofrequency lesioning that is sometimes prolonged. A needle is placed in the foramen ovale with the patient supine as previously described. The needle is advanced until spinal fluid is seen, then the patient is placed sitting at about 45 degrees. The patient's neck is flexed and 0.1–0.5 ml radio-opaque contrast is injected. Once the cistern has been demonstrated and needle position is satisfactory, the contrast is withdrawn and the same volume of glycerol is slowly injected. The patient is kept sitting for about 2 hours. This technique produces a shorter duration of analgesia than radiofrequency lesioning. It has a higher rate of recurrence of pain and although this is not always a problem in palliative care practice, it can be an issue in trigeminal neuralgia. Repeating the block may be difficult because of fibrosis in the foramen ovale.

Branches of the trigeminal nerve, such as the mandibular nerve, can be blocked more peripherally. However, the effects of a neurolytic block may be short lived and deafferentation pain may occur.

Specific complications

- Haematoma in cheek
- Facial numbness
- Dysaesthetic facial pain (anaesthesia dolorosa)
- Loss of corneal sensation
- Motor deficit after mandibular lesioning
- Carotid artery puncture
- Intrathecal injection
- Retrobulbar haematoma
- Infection
- Oculomotor weakness
- Cavernous sinus fistula
- Perioperative cardiac arrhythmias.

Brachial plexus block

There are several approaches to blocking the brachial plexus including axillary, subclavian perivascular, and interscalene techniques. The effect of a block at each level can be predicted from knowledge of the local anatomy. Each method has advantages and disadvantages. However, the axillary approach is the safest. The technique chosen depends on the experience and skill of the operator. The dose of local anaesthetic required is large for brachial blockade and the potential for adverse effects exists. Plasma local anaesthetic concentrations are similar after all three techniques.

Specific indications

- Unilateral arm pain due to malignancy such as brachial plexitis from nerve invasion[3]
- Unilateral arm pain due to treatment such as radiation plexitis
- Combined with stellate ganglion block, for arm pain with an autonomic component
- Procedures on the arm such as surgical interventions, manipulation of a dislocation, dressing changes.

Specific contraindications

- Inability to abduct the arm makes axillary block difficult
- Caution is required with axillary blockade in those with lymphoedema
- Phrenic or recurrent laryngeal nerve paralysis on the contralateral side contraindicates the interscalene approaches because of the risk of phrenic or recurrent nerve palsy on the blocked side
- Pneumothorax on the contralateral side and severe respiratory disease contraindicate the subclavian perivascular or interscalene approaches because of the risk of pneumothorax or phrenic nerve palsy on the blocked side.

Anatomy

The brachial plexus innervates the upper limb. Its roots, formed from C5, C6, C7, C8, and T1, emerge from the cervical spine between the anterior and middle scalene muscles in the neck (Fig. 7.3). The roots unite in the posterior triangle of the neck to form three trunks that pass over the first rib, lying on top of each other, superior to the subclavian artery, and behind the mid-point of the clavicle where each trunk divides into an anterior and a posterior division. The divisions form cords that pass into the axilla. These cords then give rise to the nerves that supply the arm. The intercostobrachial nerve, which is formed by branches of the intercostal nerves, supplies the skin of the axilla. This nerve is important as it is often sacrificed during axillary dissection and this commonly causes neuropathic pain in the medial aspect of the arm and the axilla. The prevertebral fascia envelops the brachial plexus from the level of the cervical vertebrae to the distal axilla, forming a subclavian perivascular space that is in continuity with the axillary perivascular space. Once a needle has entered this space, only a single injection is necessary for anaesthesia of the brachial plexus. The volume of the brachial plexus (ml) in an adult is equal to half the

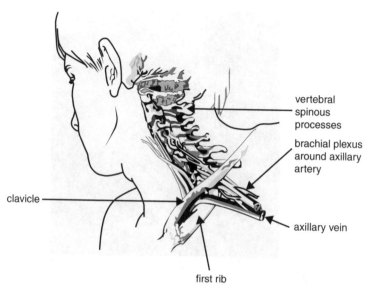

vertebral spinous processes

brachial plexus around axillary artery

clavicle

axillary vein

first rib

Fig. 7.3 Anatomy of the brachial plexus.

patients height measured in inches. The extent of the block is dependent upon the volume of local anaesthetic injected and where in the sheath the needle is placed. The use of a very large volume in the axillary block (such as 50–60 ml) extends the areas that can be covered and if the local anaesthetic is dilute then toxicity can be avoided. If motor block occurs, it is important to warn the patient and staff to protect the blocked limb until sensation returns.

Axillary block or catheterization

The patient is placed supine or sitting at 45 degrees with the arm abducted to 90 degrees and the elbow flexed. The axillary artery is palpated as high in the axilla as possible. When performing a single block, a short bevelled or pencil point 23 G or 24 G needle with an extension attached is inserted superior to the artery; cutting needles must not be used because of the risk of nerve damage. Pulsation of the needle confirms proximity to the artery, or a peripheral nerve stimulator can be used to aid needle placement (Fig. 7.4). Although the trans-arterial approach is a recognized technique, its use should be discouraged; it may result in haematoma formation and bleeding from the artery dilutes the local anaesthetic. Attempts to illicit paraesthesia

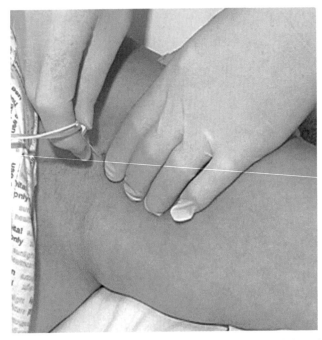

Fig. 7.4 Nerve stimulator needle placement during axillary brachial plexus block.

may result in nerve damage, but if paraesthesia occurs, this confirms proximity to the plexus. About 40 ml local anaesthetic is used—the drug and concentration chosen determine the duration and depth of the block required. Depot steroids can be injected with the local anaesthetic but there is no good evidence for efficacy. The insertion of a catheter into the brachial plexus sheath may be used to allow longer-term infusions of local anaesthetic solutions. The technique is the same as for injection, except that a larger needle is used to pass a catheter. This can be performed blindly or using fluoroscopy with contrast (Fig. 7.5). Axillary block produces reliable analgesia below the elbow; it cannot be relied upon for problems in the upper arm or shoulder. The block can take about 45 minutes to work.

Specific complications

- If larger volumes (50–60 ml) are used for axillary block, the cervical plexus may also be affected
- Nerve damage
- Intravascular injection.

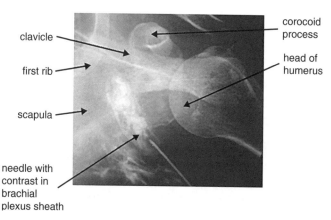

corocoid process

clavicle

head of humerus

first rib

scapula

needle with contrast in brachial plexus sheath

Fig. 7.5 X ray of injection into the sheath of the brachial plexus before catheter insertion.

Subclavian perivascular block or catheterization

The patient is placed supine with the head turned away from the side to be blocked. The lateral edge of the sternomastoid muscle is palpated just above the clavicle. Laterally, the interscalene groove is palpable and pulsation of the subclavian artery is felt as it emerges between the scalene muscles. A short, bevelled needle with an extension attached is inserted above this point and aimed caudally (Fig. 7.6). A nerve stimulator is useful

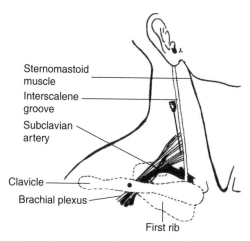

Sternomastoid muscle

Interscalene groove

Subclavian artery

Clavicle

Brachial plexus

First rib

Fig. 7.6 Subclavian perivascular brachial plexus block.

to produce paraesthesia going below the elbow. This indicates that the needle is in the correct position. A catheter can be passed into the sheath and this is easier to fix than with an axillary block. 20–40 ml local anaesthetic is injected whilst observing the patient for signs of complications. This block usually works more quickly than an axillary block. Subclavian perivascular block will produce more widespread anaesthesia and analgesic for pain or procedures on the shoulder, elbow, or arm.

Specific complications

- Pneumothorax may occur especially if the needle is directed too medially
- Phrenic nerve paralysis occurs in a third of cases and laryngeal nerve block, cervical plexus block, and sympathetic block are common
- The subclavian artery may be punctured but this reseals rapidly and does not usually cause problems.

Interscalene block or catheterization

The patient is placed supine, with the head turned away from the side to be blocked. The interscalene groove is identified as for the subclavian perivascular block. A short bevelled needle with an extension is inserted into the interscalene groove at a point level with the cricoid cartilage. A nerve stimulator can be used until paraesthesia is felt or the transverse process of the cervical vertebra is contacted (usually less than 2.5 cm from the skin) (Fig. 7.7). It is important not to direct the needle too horizontally as it may not be stopped by the transverse process, but may enter the vertebral artery, epidural space, or a dural cuff, with potentially dangerous results. 30-40 ml local anaesthetic is injected. A catheter can be passed for a longer duration of effect and is easier to fix than in the axilla. The block takes about 15 minutes to take effect. Interscalene block will produce analgesia or anaesthesia for procedures on the shoulder or arm. Block of the ulnar nerve may be delayed or absent after interscalene block, especially if less than 40 ml of local anaesthetic is used.

Specific complications

- Potential for serious adverse effects is greatest with the interscalene block. Adverse effects tend to be immediate
- The risk of pneumothorax is less after the interscalene approach than with the subclavian perivascular technique
- Vertebral artery injection

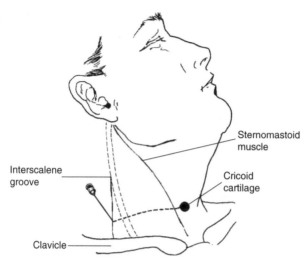

Fig. 7.7 Interscalene brachial plexus block.

- 'Total spinal' injection
- Recurrent laryngeal nerve, phrenic nerve, sympathetic and cervical plexus block are common.

Intercostal block

Intercostal blockade can be used to treat unilateral, well-localized, chest wall pain within a few dermatomes. There is a risk of pneumothorax, especially in very slim patients, in obese patients where the ribs cannot be felt or in those who have had chest surgery that may make the pleura adherent. Multiple blocks should be avoided. If several dermatomes are affected then intrapleural or paravertebral analgesia may be preferable. Local anaesthetic with or without steroid can be used. Although the effect of local anaesthetic alone is often brief, the technique may be used to provide analgesia in the acute situation, such as rib fracture. Intercostal blocks result in higher plasma local anaesthetic concentrations than any other technique because of rapid absorption from the muscle and subpleural space. It is therefore important that the toxic dose is not exceeded. Neurolytic blocks using phenol are possible, but are only really useful for anteriorly placed rib metastases. Injection into the intercostal groove posteriorly can result in spread of injectate paravertebrally. This is undesirable if a neurolytic is being used.

Specific indications

- Rib fractures
- Chest wall pain
- Rib metastases.

Specific contraindications

- Bilateral pain
- Obesity (the rib margin must be palpable if the block is to be attempted)
- Contralateral pneumothorax or pneumonectomy
- Poor respiratory function.

Anatomy

The 12 intercostal nerves are the anterior primary rami of the thoracic nerves that leave the intervertebral foramina and traverse the paravertebral space to run below each rib, together with the intercostal blood vessels. Anteriorly the neurovascular bundle runs between the external and internal intercostal muscles. The intercostal nerves are sometimes arranged as 3–4 nerve bundles rather than a single nerve. They usually run below the rib margin, but in some patients they lie above it. Each nerve gives off a lateral branch at the level of the mid-axillary line and anterior branch near the sternal edge. The upper six intercostal nerves supply the thoracic cage and the lower six nerves also supply the anterior abdominal wall. There is overlap between adjoining segments and therefore blocking a single intercostal nerve may not produce a segment of altered sensation.

Technique

The patient lies prone or in the lateral position with the side to be blocked uppermost (Fig. 7.8). The shoulder should be abducted and the arm moved forwards to move the scapula away from the angle of the upper ribs. The intercostal nerve can be blocked where the rib is palpable at the posterior costal angle at the lateral border of the sacrospinalis muscle, where the intercostal space is at its widest, or it can be blocked at the mid-axillary line (Fig. 7.9). Ideally the patient should breath-hold during the block. A 23 G short bevelled needle is inserted perpendicular to the skin and aimed slightly cephalad to strike the lower border of the chosen rib; this is uncomfortable. The needle is passed under the lower border of the rib to a depth of 3–4 mm. It is important that the patient is able to keep very still since this minimizes the risk of complications. Careful aspiration is

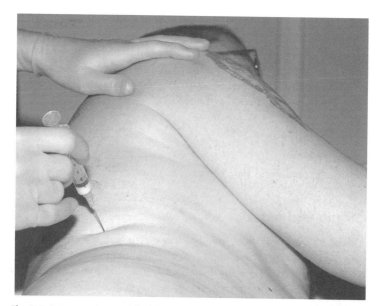

Fig. 7.8 Intercostal nerve block (point of injection demonstrated using blunt needle).

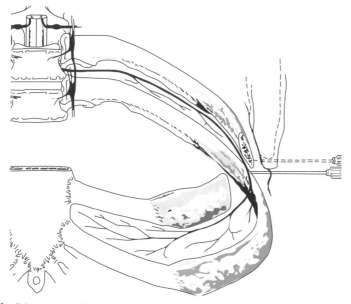

Fig. 7.9 Intercostal block.

needed to detect air or blood. The volume of drug injected determines the nature of the block. With 3–5 ml only a single level is blocked. If 20–25 ml is injected posteriorly in the chest wall, the solution spreads to enter the paravertebral and even epidural space, producing a more widespread effect including sympathetic block. Neurolytic blocks must be of small volume (0.5–1.0 ml) to produce restricted spread.

Specific complications

- Pneumothorax
- Bleeding from intercostal vessels.

Intrapleural block

Infusion of local anaesthetic into the pleural cavity can be used to provide analgesia. Injection of 20 ml local anaesthetic solution in the supine subject results in spread from the diaphragm to the lung apex and probably produces multiple intercostal, sympathetic, and perhaps splanchnic blocks.

Specific indications

- Unilateral chest wall pain over several levels such as due to malignancy, multiple rib fractures.[4]

Specific contraindications

- Bilateral pain
- Contralateral pneumothorax or pneumonectomy
- Poor respiratory function
- Inflamed chest cavity that may promote rapid local anaesthetic absorption and toxicity.

Anatomy

The pleural space extends from the lung apex to the inferior pleural reflection at about L1.

Technique

This block can be done with the patient sitting but it is usually more comfortable if the patient lies on their side with the affected side uppermost.

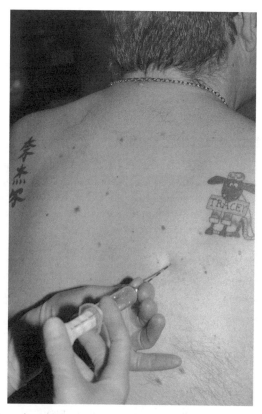

Fig. 7.10 Intrapleural injection. Loss of resistance technique.

Local anaesthetic is infiltrated superior to the 8th rib in the 7th intercostal space about 10 cm lateral to the spinous processes. A needle that will allow passage of a catheter (usually an epidural needle) is attached to a syringe of saline and advanced over the top of the rib using a loss of resistance technique (Fig. 7.10). When the pleural cavity is entered the saline solution injects easily. Another technique is to remove the syringe barrel and observe the falling column of saline when the pleural cavity is entered. A catheter is then threaded about 10 cm intrapleurally, avoiding the entry of air. The catheter may be tunnelled subcutaneously if it is to be used long term. Analgesia may be achieved by injection boluses of 20–30 ml local anaesthetic or by infusion, taking care not to exceed the recommended maximum daily dose.

Specific complications

- Pneumothorax
- Bleeding from intercostal vessels
- Horner's syndrome
- Patchy analgesia.

Paravertebral block

Spinal nerves can be blocked at any level as they emerge from the vertebral foramina. In the cervical or thoracic region the block should only be performed unilaterally because of the risk of complications with bilateral blocks (phrenic nerve palsy, pneumothorax). In the lumbar region bilateral paravertebral block is possible.

Specific indications

- Pain in a limited dermatomal distribution in the cervical, thoracic, or lumbar region
- Nerve invasion from tumour
- Radicular pain from spinal degeneration
- Radicular pain from vertebral collapse (metastasis or osteoporosis).

Specific contraindications

- Cervical and thoracic blocks in patients with respiratory compromise.

Anatomy

Cadaver and radiographic studies have demonstrated considerable variability in the dimensions of the paravertebral spaces. There is highly variable spread of injected solutions that may track over several segments, into the pleural cavity and also epidurally. The use of fluoroscopy is recommended for this technique. The use of neurolytic in this area has fallen out of favour because of the risk of significant complications such as paraplegia even after relatively small volumes have been used.

Technique

The precise method of injection depends on the spinal level in question. The basic technique involves visualizing the vertebral transverse process at the level to be blocked using fluoroscopy, and advancing a short, bevelled

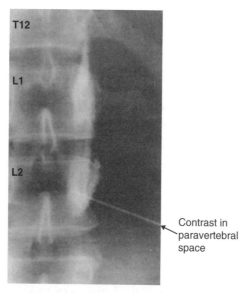

Contrast in
paravertebral
space

Fig. 7.11 Antero-posterior view of paravertebral block in the lumbar region.

needle to contact it. The needle is then redirected caudally to a depth of
1–2 cm so that it lies near the nerve root. Radio-opaque contrast is then
used to check the needle position before about 5 ml of local anaesthetic
with or without steroid is injected (Fig. 7.11).

Specific complications

- Neural damage
- In the cervical region, phrenic and recurrent laryngeal nerve block
- In the thorax, pneumothorax
- Sympathetic block
- Total spinal.

Lumbar psoas compartment block

It is possible to block the lumbar plexus where it passes via the psoas compartment and this provides analgesia for the hip and leg.[5] The technique
is simple and safe. A single injection of local anaesthetic and steroid can be
used—or an infusion of local anaesthetic can provide a more prolonged
effect.

Specific indications

- Unilateral pain in the hip or leg, such as hip pain from fracture or metastases
- Lumbar nerve root invasion in the region of the psoas muscle.

Specific contraindications

- Pain that arises more proximally in the nervous system will not be helped by lumbar psoas block
- Bilateral pain is usually better managed by spinal techniques
- Pain in the lower leg and foot is not usually well managed
- This block does not routinely affect the sacral plexus and obturator nerves. Therefore pain transmitted via these may not be amenable to lumbar plexus block.

Anatomy

The lower limb is supplied by the lumbosacral plexus formed from the anterior primary rami of L2-S3. The L1-4 nerve roots emerge from vertebral foramina and enter the psoas muscle where the lumbar plexus is usually formed; this muscle is enclosed in a sheath that confines the spread of anaesthetic solution placed at L3. The L5 root emerges below the origin of the psoas muscle; it lies within the space between psoas and quadratus lumborum. Local anaesthetic injected here still bathes the lumbar plexus. The sacral nerve roots are not blocked using this technique.

Technique

The patient lies on their side with the side to be treated uppermost. The success of the block is improved by the use of fluoroscopy. A needle of at least 15 cm is usually needed to reach the transverse process and if a catheter technique is to be used then a long epidural type needle is needed. The L4 vertebral transverse process is identified and the needle is advanced to contact it. The needle is then partly withdrawn and directed cephalad until it slides past the transverse process as detected by loss of resistance to air. Confirmation of needle position by the use of radio-opaque contrast is useful (Fig. 7.12). A nerve stimulator can also be used to display quadriceps contractions that signify correct needle placement. About 30 ml solution can be used to provide a single block.[6] If a catheter technique is to be used it is useful to inject 20–30 ml saline to distend the space before

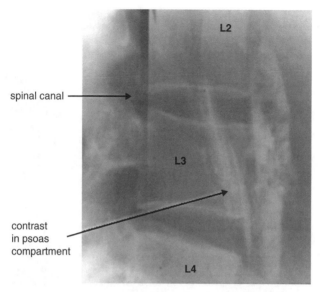

spinal canal

contrast
in psoas
compartment

Fig. 7.12 Lateral view of psoas compartment block. Contrast flows diagonally across the vertebra within the psoas sheath. Contrast has been also placed anterior to the vertebra and behind the aorta to show the distinction between psoas block and the more anterior sympathetic block.

threading a 7–10 cm catheter. Long-term catheters should be tunnelled subcutaneously.

Specific complications

- Damage to lumbosacral plexus
- Psoas abscess
- Paravertebral and epidural spread of injectate
- Sympathetic block and hypotension.

Epidural or caudal block

Single epidural or caudal injections of local anaesthetic and steroid can be used to treat a variety of conditions (Fig. 7.13). Epidural steroids are probably effective in the short term for lumbar, non-cancer, radicular pain.

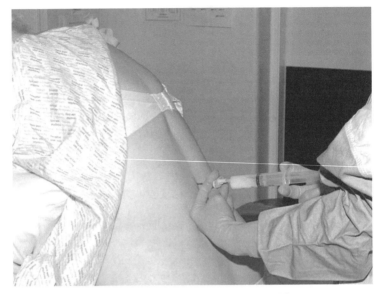

Fig. 7.13 Epidural injection of local anaesthetic and steroid.

There is little evidence for their use in malignant nerve root pain, however many case reports and series suggest good results. Single epidural injections are simple and relatively safe.

Specific indications

- Back pain due to vertebral problems such as metastases, osteoporotic collapse
- Coccydynia
- Unilateral or bilateral leg pain such as radicular pain from degeneration or malignancy.

Specific contraindications

- Local or systemic infection
- Uncorrectable co-aggulopathy
- Raised intracranial pressure
- Impending spinal cord or cauda equina compression.

Anatomy, techniques, and specific complications (see Chapter 8)

Intrathecal neurolytic injection of sacrococcygeal nerve roots

Intrathecal neurolysis using a single injection can destroy sensory nerve roots at any spinal level. In the past it was commonly used for unilateral pain in the thoracic and lumbar area. Serious adverse effects such as motor blockade are possible and now with the advent of spinal drug delivery (Chapter 8) this technique is not used commonly. However, intrathecal neurolysis still has value in the management of some pain problems such as pelvic and perineal pain.[7, 8] Neurolysis is a simple procedure that can be carried out in elderly and debilitated patients. The object is to deposit tiny amounts of phenol accurately onto the target nerves. The block can last for many months and can be repeated if necessary. It is often useful to perform a preliminary predictive test dose using local anaesthetic.

Specific indications

- Pain affecting a limited number of dermatomes (sacral and coccygeal segments are the most appropriate)
- Perineal or rectal pain such as that from vulval tumours or fungating rectal tumours
- Patients who already have a urinary catheter and stoma do not risk incontinence but autonomic nerve problems are not an inevitable consequence of the block
- Good response to an intrathecal test dose of local anaesthetic.

Specific contraindications

- Local or systemic infection
- Uncorrectable co-aggulopathy
- Raised intracranial pressure
- Impending spinal cord or cauda equina compression.

Anatomy (see Chapter 8)

Technique

The procedure is performed with the patient sitting with the spine flexed. If the patient cannot sit then analgesia may be needed. Heavy sedation should not be used as the patient must remain sitting and it is important to maintain co-operation. Needle size and placement, positioning the patient, and injection should be identical for test dosing and neurolysis. A 20 G spinal needle is introduced intrathecally at the L5/S1 junction (Fig. 7.14). The needle needs to be large enough to allow injection of viscous neurolytic solution. The patient is leaned backwards over the edge of the trolley at an angle of about 45 degrees and supported by at least two assistants. The spinal needle is then very slowly withdrawn until spinal fluid just drips from the needle, indicating that it is placed in the posterior part of the sub-arachnoid space. The aim is to apply neurolytic to the posteriorly placed sensory nerve roots and spare autonomic and motor pathways. Injection of 0.6 ml 0.5% hyperbaric bupivacaine can be used as a test dose. For neurolysis, injection of hyperbaric 0.6 ml 6% phenol in glycerine is performed over 2 minutes. The injection needs to be slow to prevent jetting of solution anteriorly onto the motor nerve roots. After injection the patient is meticulously kept leaning back at 45 degrees and then carefully rotated to

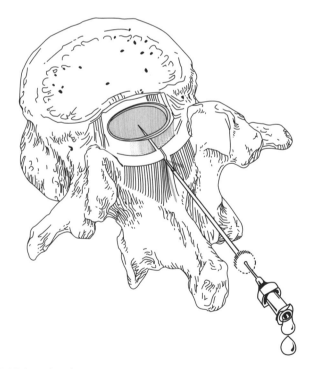

Fig. 7.14 Intrathecal puncture.

maintain this position on the trolley supported by pillows. The patient must remain in this position for at least half an hour and preferably for a few hours to allow the phenol to fix to the posterior (sensory) nerve roots and avoid any motor blockade. The local anaesthetic effect of the phenol usually means that the underlying pain will have abated, so the patient should be comfortable. The full neurolytic effect may not be manifest for 24–48 hours.

Specific complications

- Spinal headache
- Problems with bladder and/or bowel control
- Erectile and other sexual dysfunction
- Cauda equina trauma from the spinal needle.

Autonomic blocks

Sphenopalatine ganglion block

This block can be used in managing head and neck pain from a variety of causes. Local anaesthetic has been used to treat acute migraine, cluster headaches, and a variety of facial neuralgias. The use of neurolytic in this area can be hazardous because of the local anatomical relations of the ganglion.

Specific indications

- Pain from head and neck cancer.[9, 10]

Specific contraindications

- Caution in patients with postural hypotension.

Anatomy

The sphenopalatine ganglion is a large collection of neurones located in the pterygopalatine fossa, posterior to the middle turbinate. A thin layer of connective tissue and mucous membrane covers it. It receives its sensory supply from the trigeminal nerve, motor supply from the facial nerve, and sympathetic input from the carotid plexus. Its efferent branches supply the orbit, inside of the nose, gums, palate, and some of the throat.

Technique

The sphenopalatine ganglion can be blocked topically via the nasal membranes or by injection via the greater palatine foramen in the hard palate.

Specific complications

- Epistaxis
- Hypotension

Stellate ganglion block

The sympathetic nerve supply to the head, neck, and arm can be interrupted at the stellate ganglion to produce vasodilatation and analgesia for some conditions. Single or repeated injections are usually performed. Catheter techniques have been tried, but the catheters are difficult to fix and tend to migrate. Neurolytic stellate ganglion block carries a risk of serious complications due to its anatomical relationships (see below).

Specific indications

- Pain affecting the head or arm that has an autonomic component, such as head and neck tumour, Pancoasts tumour
- Refractory angina that does not respond to medical management
- Acute herpes zoster affecting the head.

Specific contraindications

- Caution in patients with severe cardio-respiratory problems
- Simultaneous bilateral blocks should be avoided as bilateral phrenic or recurrent laryngeal nerve block may occur.

Anatomy

The stellate ganglion is formed by fusion of the inferior cervical ganglion with the upper thoracic ganglion. The sympathetic chain travels upwards from the thorax, crosses the neck of the first rib and ascends to the skull base embedded in the posterior wall of the carotid sheath. The sympathetic chain is anterior to the fascia covering the prevertebral muscles in the neck that form a thin layer over the transverse processes of the cervical vertebrae. The transverse process of the sixth cervical vertebra is an important landmark for this block that can be palpated laterally at the level of the cricoid cartilage. The stellate ganglion lies very close to many important structures that must be considered during injection.

- The carotid sheath is anterior to the sympathetic chain
- The pharynx, oesophagus, and larynx are medial and the recurrent laryngeal nerve runs between them

- The vertebral artery runs upwards—it is enclosed in foramina in the transverse processes
- Cervical spinal nerves pass out between the transverse processes encased in long dural sleeves
- The dome of the pleura is inferior to the stellate ganglion.

Technique

Stellate ganglion block is performed by injection of local anaesthetic into the correct tissue plane with the patient supine or sitting at 45 degrees (Fig. 7.15).

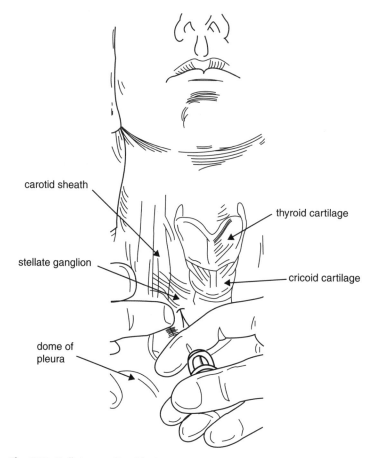

Fig. 7.15 Stellate ganglion block.

The extent of the block is partly dependant upon the volume of drug injected and the patient's position; small volumes block the head and neck whilst larger volumes also block the arm, especially if the patient is sitting during the block. Some operators use fluoroscopy with radio-opaque contrast to facilitate needle placement. The transverse process of C6 is palpated at, or slightly above, the level of the cricoid cartilage and carotid pulsation is felt laterally. The needle is inserted at right angles to the skin to strike the transverse process of C6. If the needle passes too deeply then it may enter the vertebral artery or dural sleeve, or produce tingling in the arm by impinging on the brachial plexus. It is vital that local anaesthetic is not injected unless the operator is sure that the needle is anterior to the transverse process. 10–20 ml of 0.25–0.5% plain local anaesthetic is used to achieve a prolonged effect. Physical signs of a correctly placed injection include miosis, enophthalmos, ptosis, suffusion of the conjunctiva, blocked nose, dry warm skin, and flushing on the side of injection. However, signs in the head do not confirm that the arm has also been successfully blocked.

Specific complications

- Carotid puncture with haematoma
- Recurrent laryngeal nerve block occurs in 10% patients and produces hoarseness. Patients should eat or drink cautiously for several hours afterwards. Swallowing should be assessed with cool water first
- Brachial plexus block
- Phrenic nerve block
- Intravascular injection will produce a severe and rapid toxic reaction, as the vertebral artery will carry local anaesthetic directly to the brain
- Aspiration prior to injection cannot guarantee that the needle is not subarachnoid as the dura can act like a flap valve on the end of the needle. Injection into a dural sleeve will produce a 'total spinal'
- Pleural puncture and pneumothorax are potential problems if the needle is either sited too low or directed caudad
- Osteitis and mediastinitis may occur after oesophageal puncture.

Coeliac plexus block (CPB) and greater splanchnic nerve block

Blocking the coeliac plexus interrupts the autonomic supply to the upper gastrointestinal tract and provides good quality analgesia. CBP is performed with the patient lying prone, and usually requires sedation or anaesthesia.

Patients must be relatively robust to undergo the procedure so CPB should not be used as a treatment of last resort. The potential complications of the procedure can be serious and these must be fully discussed with the patient. Based on data from uncontrolled trials, neurolytic CPB is an effective analgesic method for pain associated with pancreatic and non-pancreatic intra-abdominal malignancies; it may be associated with prolonged survival.[11–13] A diagnostic block with local anaesthetic can be used as a prelude to a neurolytic block with alcohol. However this does not always predict success.[14] Approximately 90% patients achieve at least partial pain relief for three months and beyond. Assessment of short-term analgesic efficacy in 18 trials of CPB (989 patients) showed that 89% had at least partial relief and of these, 59% had experienced complete relief by two weeks. Long-term efficacy was assessed in 273 patients; 90% experienced at least partial relief at three months or beyond. Six trials (53 patients) reported that 73–92% had at least partial relief of pain until the time of death.[15]

Indications

- Pain associated with upper abdominal cancer from structures proximal to the splenic flexure such as primary stomach, biliary or pancreatic tumours, and liver metastases. There is no evidence that those with pancreatic cancer fare any better or worse than those with other upper gastrointestinal tumours.

- Intractable nausea that does not respond to routine therapies.

Specific contraindications

- Pain due to tumour invasion of the posterior abdominal wall is not usually helped by CPB

- Patients with extensive spread of tumour around the coeliac plexus may not achieve good analgesia because of limited spread of the neurolytic[16]

- Very debilitated patients may not be able to tolerate the procedure

- Dehydrated patients may become hypotensive after CPB

- Caution in patients who are sexually active as sexual dysfunction may occur.

Anatomy

The coeliac plexus consists of large, paired ganglia situated in the upper abdomen (Fig. 7.16). The size and exact position of the coeliac ganglia is slightly variable; the left is usually lower than the right. The coeliac plexus arises from the sympathetic fibres of the splanchnic nerves from T5-T12.

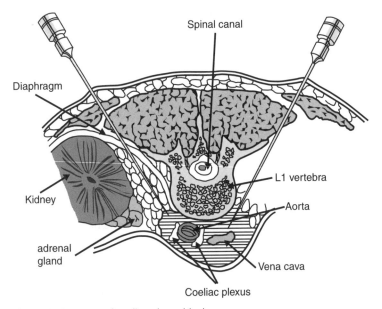

Fig. 7.16 Anatomy of coeliac plexus block.

It contains preganglionic afferent fibres, parasympathetic preganglionic fibres, and postganglionic sympathetic fibres. Pain is transmitted from the upper abdomen—pancreas, diaphragm, liver, spleen, small bowel, ascending and proximal transverse colon, adrenal glands, abdominal aorta, and mesentery. Large bowel distal to the splenic flexure and the pelvic organs send visceral sympathetic nerves via the hypogastric plexus. Therefore, a CPB does not completely denervate the viscera. The coeliac plexus lies in loose areolar tissues within the retroperitoneal space posterior to the stomach and the pancreas and close to the coeliac artery. It overlaps the aorta at the level of the L1 vertebra. The plexus is separated from the vertebrae by the crus of the diaphragm that originates from the anterolateral surfaces of the upper lumbar vertebrae. The tendinous origins of the diaphragm blend with the anterior longitudinal vertebral ligaments. This forms an important barrier to the spread of injectate.

Techniques

All patients require intravenous fluids during and after the CPB. They should wear support stockings to try to reduce postural hypotension. Vital signs must be monitored throughout and after the procedure. Supplementary oxygen is usually given during the block, especially if the patient has chest problems that may be exacerbated by lying prone. Many different techniques have been described for CPB with different needle approaches, solutions, and radiological guidance, such as fluoroscopy, CT, or MR scanning and ultrasound (Figs. 7.17 and 7.18).[11, 17] There is no evidence that any technique has significant advantages over the others. In view of this it would seem best that each clinician uses the technique with which he is most comfortable.

Retro-crural CPB. The patient lies prone and the L1 vertebra is identified radiologically. The skin is infiltrated generously with local anaesthetic bilaterally, just below the 12th rib and about 7 cm from the midline. Needles are inserted and aimed cephalad to strike the lateral border of L1. The needles are then walked off the anterior border of the vertebral body to lie about 1–2 cm anteriorly. The right-sided needle usually needs to be more anterior than the left. The needle position is checked radiologically in both planes, and a small volume of radio-opaque contrast is injected. The contrast should spread mainly cephalad, into the retro-aortic space, in front of, and lateral to, the lower thoracic and L1 vertebra. Then about 10 ml local anaesthetic is injected into each needle and time is allowed for this to take effect. Sedation may also be given prior to injection of 25–40 ml

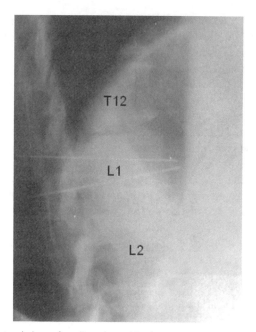

Fig. 7.17 Lateral view of coeliac plexus block.

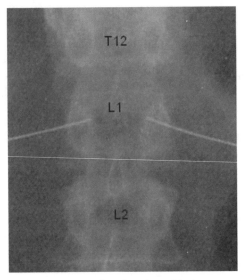

Fig. 7.18 Antero-posterior view of coeliac plexus block.

alcohol (50–100%) on each side. This produces a classic splanchnic nerve block. The neurolytic solution spreads to the retro-aortic coeliac fibres and rostrally to the splanchnic nerves. Some solution may go downwards towards the ganglia via the aortic hiatus in the diaphragm.

Trans-crural CPB. This technique is performed in a similar way to the retro-crural block. It involves advancing the needles 1–2 cm more anteriorly. The needles pass through the crura, when loss of resistance may be felt. The needles should then lie anterolateral to the aorta near the coeliac ganglia. Injection of radio-opaque contrast shows linear spread around the aorta. A similar volume of neurolytic (25–40 ml) is used. A single needle technique with unilateral left-sided injection has been described where the needle is placed more anterior to the aorta. However with this approach, even if 50 ml of neurolytic solution is used, the spread is not as great as with 25 ml injected on each side.

Trans-aortic CPB. A single needle is introduced from the left side to pass through the aorta until no further blood can be aspirated. This means that the needle lies just anterior to the aorta close to the coeliac plexus. Contrast spreads in the pre-aortic areolar tissue. Smaller volumes 15–30 ml of neurolytic can be used, as the needle is closer to the plexus. This may be less reliable if there is para-aortic lymphadenopathy that might limit the spread of solutions.

Anterior CPB. The patient can lie supine for this approach. The needle is introduced through the epigastrium to reach the L1 vertebra and then withdrawn 1–1.5 cm under ultrasound guidance. The needle is positioned just anterior to the diaphragmatic crus at the level of the coeliac artery. Smaller volumes (15–30 ml) of neurolytic are needed with this approach. Assessment of an anterior CPB technique using CT guidance at 30 days after the block showed that spread of neurolytic into three or four quadrants around the coeliac plexus is needed to achieve good analgesia. Distortion of local anatomy due to tumour spread resulted in adequate spread of neurolytic and good analgesia in only 28% cases.[18]

Intra-operative CPB. During surgery it is possible to inject neurolytic solutions retro-peritoneally into the area where the splanchnic nerves join the coeliac plexus. This can provide good analgesia for patients with pancreatic tumour and one prospective study has shown prolonged survival after this type of CPB. However, there are some difficulties with this approach as the needle may not be easy to place and dissection may impair the spread of injectate. The success rate may be lower than with the percutaneous approach.

Greater splanchnic nerve block. This technique involves placing needles more cephalad to lie at the anterolateral surface of the T12 vertebral body. Needles are inserted 3–4 cm lateral to the midline just below the 12th rib. The risk of pneumothorax is greater than with most other approaches. Smaller volumes (8–10 ml) of neurolytic solution can be used; therefore phenol 8% should be used rather than alcohol. There are no comparative studies to compare this block with more classical approaches to the coeliac plexus.

Specific complications

- Local pain in 96% cases.

- Diarrhoea in 44% of patients. This usually resolves within 48 hours but may persist. Octreotide may be helpful if this becomes troublesome.

- Hypotension in 38% that usually improves within 48 hours. Adequate hydration and elastic stockings help in most cases. Occasionally vasopressors are needed.

- Acute alcohol intoxication has been seen.

- More severe effects were reported in 13 trials. Neurological complications such as lower extremity weakness and paraesthesia, lumbar plexus injection, epidural anaesthesia, and lumbar puncture were reported in 1% of patients. Incontinence and sexual dysfunction can occur. Paraplegia may occur—perhaps due to anterior spinal artery compromise.

- Significant non-neurological adverse effects, including pneumothorax, shoulder, chest and pleuritic pain, hiccuping, and haematuria occurred in a further 1% of patients. Aortic dissection and silent gastric perforation have been reported.

- Decreased complication rates may be expected when trans-aortic or anterior approaches are used because smaller volumes of neurolytic are needed. There is however no trial evidence to support this.

Lumbar sympathetic block

Sympathetic denervation of the whole lower limb requires blockade of the 2nd, 3rd, and 4th lumbar ganglia.

Specific indications

- Unilateral or bilateral ischaemic leg pain
- Pain mediated via the sympathetic nervous system[19]
- Bilateral sympathectomy for rectal tenesmus.[20]

Specific contraindications

- Unilateral block can lead to sexual problems and this is even more likely with bilateral block. This should be carefully considered in sexually active patients.

Anatomy

The sympathetic chain is anterolateral to the vertebral bodies on the psoas muscle in the retroperitoneal tissues. The genitofemoral nerve is slightly lateral. The aorta and inferior vena cava lie anteriorly, and the kidney and ureter are posterolateral.

Technique

The patient lies on their side with the affected limb uppermost. Using the single needle technique a 15 cm needle is inserted 9–12 cm from the midline, level with L3. The needle is advanced until it makes contact with the lateral aspect of the L3 vertebral body, confirmed by fluoroscopy (Fig. 7.19). There may be a loss of resistance as the needle passes through the anterior aspect of the psoas fascia. Lateral fluoroscopy should show the needle point level with the front of the vertebra. Anteroposterior fluoroscopy should show the needle about 25% of the way across the vertebra. The needle position should be confirmed using radio-opaque contrast that should be seen

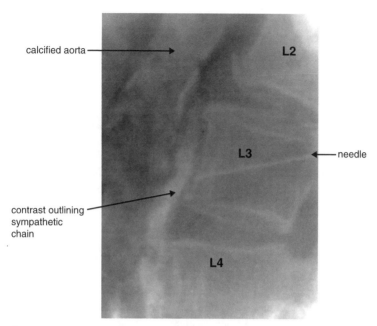

Fig. 7.19 Lateral view of lumbar sympathectomy single needle technique.

as a narrow strip in front of the vertebrae, not spreading anteriorly (suggesting intra-peritoneal injection) or posteriorly (suggesting spread towards somatic nerves) or within psoas. Either 6–8 ml local anaesthetic or 8% aqueous phenol should be injected. The local anaesthetic effect of phenol is usually seen within minutes but the neurolytic effect may not be fully manifest for 48 hours. Some operators place three needles at L2, L3, and L4 and inject smaller volumes of neurolytic at each site. There are no good comparative studies of single versus multiple needle techniques. Radiofrequency lesioning can also be used to ablate the sympathetic chain.

Specific complications

- Postural hypotension, especially if bilateral block is performed
- Genitofemoral neuritis leading to thigh pain
- Sexual dysfunction
- Damage to kidney or ureter
- Injection into lumbar psoas muscle causing damage to lumbar plexus with leg pain, altered sensation, and motor block

- Injection into the aortic wall leading to dissection
- Intra-peritoneal injection
- Epidural or intrathecal injection has been described.

Superior hypogastric plexus block

Pain arising from the viscera and somatic structures within the pelvis and perineum may be treated by neurolytic block of the hypogastric plexus. If diagnostic block is performed prior to neurolytic block and only positive responders are treated, then over 70% patients achieve at least 50% pain relief for at least 3 weeks with greater than 40% reduction in opioid requirement. The block can be repeated successfully.[21]

Specific indications

- Pelvic pain due to gynaecological, distal gut, or urological malignancy.

Specific contraindications

- The procedure must be carefully considered in sexually active patients because of the risk of sexual dysfunction
- Extensive tumour spread within the pelvis may limit the spread of neurolytic.

Anatomy

The superior hypogastric plexus is an extension of the pre-aortic plexus; it receives fibres from the lumbar sympathetic nerve of L5 and contains mainly sympathetic fibres. It is situated at the level of the L5/S1 disc. It lies close to the sympathetic chain, with the iliac arteries and ureters lying lateral to it. It passes distally to form the hypogastric nerve that connects with the inferior hypogastric plexus. The hypogastric plexus and nerves are associated with the major blood vessels and so, like the aorta, they lie slightly to the left.

Technique

The block is performed with the patient lying prone. The L4/5 spinous processes are identified and a needle is inserted on the left about 7 cm from the midline. It is directed caudally under fluoroscopy to lie at the anterior junction of L5/S1; it should be less than 1 cm anterior to it. Needle position is confirmed with radio-opaque contrast and 4–6 ml of 8% phenol is

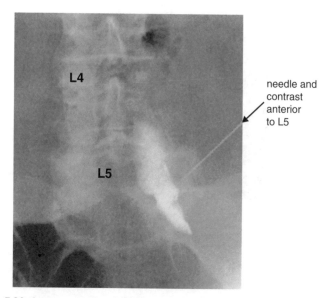

needle and
contrast
anterior
to L5

Fig. 7.20 Antero-posterior view of superior hypogastric plexus block.

injected (Fig. 7.20). Some operators use bilateral needling. The plexus can also be ablated with radiofrequency lesioning.

Specific complications
- Lumbar nerve root damage.

Presacral ganglion impar block

Pain arising from the viscera and somatic structures within the pelvis and perineum may be improved by neurolytic block of the ganglion impar (ganglion of Walther).[22, 23]

Specific indications
- Pelvic pain due to gynaecological, distal gut, or urological malignancy
- Perineal pain.

Specific contraindication
- Perineal infection or ulceration may increase the risk of infection.

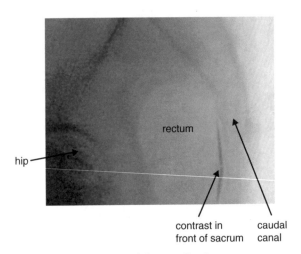

Fig. 7.21 Lateral view of injection of the ganglion impar.

Anatomy

The ganglion impar is the most caudal ganglion of the sympathetic trunk. It is usually formed by the fusion of the ganglia from both sides and it lies in the midline anterior to the sacrococcygeal junction.

Technique

The block can be done with the patient lying in the lateral, prone, or lithotomy position. A spinal needle, bent to an angle of 30 degrees, is inserted via the anococcygeal ligament and advanced under fluoroscopy until the tip is located in the retro-peritoneum at the level of the sacrococcygeal junction. Needle position is confirmed with radio-opaque contrast and 4–6 ml of 8% phenol is injected (Fig. 7.21).

Specific complications

• Rectal puncture
• Injection of neurolytic into nerve roots leading to neuritis.

Further reading

Brown DL (1999). *Atlas of regional anesthesia*, 2nd edn. W B Saunders Company, Philadelphia, PA.

Hahn MB, McQuillan PM, and Sheplock GJ (1996). *Regional anaesthesia: an atlas of anatomy and techniques*. Mosby, St Louis, MO.

Raj PP, Lou L, Erdine S, *et al.* (2003). *Radiographic imaging for regional anaesthesia and Pain management.* Churchill Livingstone, Edinburgh.

References

1. Shapshay SM, Scott RM, McCann CF, *et al.* (1980). Pain control in advanced and recurrent head and neck cancer. *Otolaryngol Clin North Am* **13**:551–60.
2. Sist T and Wong C (2000). Difficult problems and their solutions in patients with cancer pain of the head and neck areas. *Curr Rev Pain* **4**:206–14.
3. Vranken JH, Zuurmond WW, and de Lange JJ (2000). Continuous brachial plexus block as treatment for the Pancoast syndrome. *Clin J Pain* **16**:327–33.
4. Waldman SD, Allen ML, and Cronen MC (1989). Subcutaneous tunnelled intrapleural catheters in the long-term relief of right upper quadrant pain of malignant origin. *J Pain Symptom Manage* **4**:86–9.
5. Chayen D, Nathan H, and Chayen M (1976). The psoas compartment block. *Anesthesiology* **45**:95–9.
6. Parkinson SK, Mueller JB, Little WLL, *et al.* (1989). Extent of blockade with various approaches to the lumbar plexus. *Anesth Analg* **68**:243–8.
7. Rodriguez-Bigas M, Petrelli NJ, Herrera L, *et al.* (1991). Intrathecal phenol rhizotomy for management of pain in recurrent unresectable carcinoma of the rectum. *Surg Gynecol Obstet* **173**:41–4.
8. Slatkin NE and Rhiner M (2003). Phenol saddle blocks for intractable pain at end of life: report of four cases and literature review. *Am J Hosp Pall Care* **20**:62–6.
9. Varghese BT, Koshy RC, Sebastian P, *et al.* (2002). Combined sphenopalatine ganglion and mandibular nerve, neurolytic block for pain due to advanced head and neck cancer. *Palliat Med* **16**:447–8.
10. Prasanna A and Murthy PS (1993). Sphenopalatine ganglion block and pain of cancer. *J Pain Symptom Manage* **8**:125.
11. Mercadante S and Nicosia F (1998). Celiac plexus block: a reappraisal. *Reg Anesth Pain Med* **23**:37–48.
12. Kawamata M, Ishitani K, Ishikawa K, *et al.* (1996). A comparison between celiac plexus block and morphine treatment on quality of life in patients with pancreatic cancer. *Pain* **64**:597–602.
13. Staats P, Hekmat H, Sauter P, *et al.* (2001) The effects of alcohol celiac plexus block, pain and mood on longevity in patients with unresectable pancreatic cancer: a double blind, randomised, placebo-controlled study. *Pain Med* **2**:28–34.
14. Yuen TS, Ng KF, and Tsui SL (2002). Neurolytic celiac plexus block for visceral abdominal malignancy: is prior diagnostic block warranted? *Anesth Intensive Care* **30**:442–8.

15. Eisenberg E, Carr DB, and Chalmers TC (1995). Neurolytic celiac plexus block for treatment of cancer pain: a meta-analysis. *Anesth Analg* **80**:290–5.

16. De Cicco M, Matovic M, Bortolussi R, *et al.* (2001). Celiac plexus block: injectate spread and pain relief in patients with regional anatomic distortions. *Anesthesiology* **94**:561–5.

17 Ischia S, Ischia A, Polati E, *et al.* (1992). Three posterior percutaneous celiac block techniques. *Anesthesiology* **76**:534–40.

18. Cariati M, De Martini G, Pretolesi F, *et al.* (2002). CT-guided superior hypogastric plexus block. *J Comput Assist Tomogr* **26**:428–31.

19. de Leon-Casasola OA (2000). Critical evaluation of chemical neurolysis of the sympathetic axis for cancer pain. *Cancer Control* **7**:142–8.

20. Bristow A and Foster JM (1988). Lumbar sympathectomy in the management of rectal tenesmoid pain. *Ann R Coll Surg Engl* **70**:38–9.

21. Plancarte R, de Leon-Casasola OA, El-Helaly M, *et al.* (1997). Neurolytic superior hypogastric plexus block for chronic pelvic pain associated with cancer. *Reg Anesth* **22**:562–8.

22. Plancarte R, Amescua C, and Patt RB (1990). Presacral blockade of the ganglion of Walther. *Anesthesiology* **73**:A751.

23. Wilsey C, Ashford NS, and Dolin SJ (2002). Presacral neurolytic block for relief of pain from pelvic cancer: description and use of a CT-guided lateral approach. *Palliat Med* **16**:441–4.

8

Spinal drug delivery

Spinal drug delivery was suggested more than 25 years ago when opioid receptors were discovered in the spinal cord. The term spinal drug delivery includes both epidural and intrathecal routes. It offers excellent analgesia and can reduce the burden of drug side-effects as analgesics are infused directly to receptors with relatively small doses reaching the systemic circulation. However, this technique should only be considered when simpler, safer, and more economical methods have been tried and failed. Fewer than 2% of patients with pain from cancer are candidates for spinal drug delivery. Both careful patient selection and education of patients and health care professionals are crucial.[1, 2] Detailed explanation of the benefits and burdens is required before patients can take the decision to embark upon this treatment. It is important that patient, carer, and staff expectations are realistic. All spinal systems should be cared for according to strict local guidelines to optimize analgesia and minimize adverse events.[3] The need for good community support should not be underestimated; for most patients the majority of their care should be provided at home.

There is some preliminary evidence that intrathecal drug delivery (ITDD) may improve survival.[4] In a multicentre, randomized controlled trial, 202 patients with refractory cancer pain were randomized to receive either comprehensive medical management (CMM) or CMM and ITDD. Patients could cross over from CMM to ITDD if pain control was a problem. Pain and drug toxicity were assessed. ITDD produced better pain control and fewer side-effects than CMM alone. Survival was improved in the ITDD group (54%) compared with the CMM group (37%) at 6 months. As survival was not a primary end point in this study design, further work is needed to elucidate this issue.

Practical anatomy of the spinal canal

A thorough working knowledge of spinal anatomy is essential for all practitioners involved in caring for patients receiving spinal drugs. It is

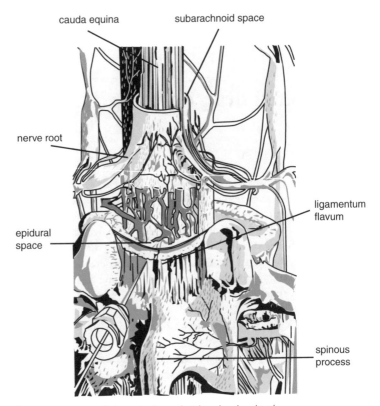

Fig. 8.1 Anatomy of the spinal canal at low lumbar level.

important that all grades of staff understand the distinction between *intrathecal* (subarachnoid) drug delivery into cerebrospinal fluid (CSF) and *epidural* drug administration into the more superficial epidural space (Fig. 8.1). Drug doses and the risks of some complications differ greatly between these two routes.

Intrathecal drug delivery (ITDD)

There are 31 pairs of spinal nerves (8 cervical, 12 thoracic, 5 lumbar, 5 sacral, and 1 coccygeal). The upper 7 cervical nerves emerge above their same-numbered vertebral bodies, C8 emerges between C7 and T1 and the remaining roots emerge below their same-numbered vertebrae.

Membranes and CSF surround the brain, spinal cord, and nerve roots. The total volume of CSF in an adult is approximately 120 ml. The CSF around the brain is continuous with that in the spinal canal via the foramen magnum and therefore any spinal intrathecal drugs have direct access to the brain stem and higher centres.

Intrathecal injection can be performed from cervical to lumbar levels. The dura terminates at a variable level, usually at S2 in adults, but in some cases reaching S4/5 (the dura extends more caudally in children). It is therefore possible accidentally to enter the subarachnoid space during caudal epidural injection. It is preferable to perform any injection below L2 where the spinal cord normally terminates in an adult; this reduces the risk of direct spinal cord damage. However, intrathecal injection may be required nearer the dermatome where pain originates. The smallest practicable intrathecal needle should be used to reduce the leakage of CSF and thus the incidence of headache. Spinal injection is safest when the patient is awake so that they can alert the practitioner to pain or paraesthesia that might indicate neural trauma. However, it is not always possible to perform these techniques in a conscious patient, as getting and maintaining the patient in a suitable position may be too painful.

Epidural drug delivery

Epidural injection or cannulation can be performed at any level from cervical to sacral; different levels require slightly different techniques and have different risks and benefits. Unlike ITDD, the site of analgesia produced by an epidural infusion depends on the level chosen for injection or catheterization and the volume of solution infused. The epidural space is largely a potential space, bounded superiorly where the periosteal and spinal layers of the dura fuse at the foramen magnum. Therefore drugs injected epidurally do not usually pass intracranially, although large volumes injected into the cervical epidural space may spread further than anticipated. The epidural space continues inferiorly to the sacrococcygeal membrane where it is entered during caudal epidural block. The lateral limits of the epidural space are formed by the vertebral pedicles and intervertebral foramina and injectate will flow out of the foramina into the paravertebral spaces (Fig. 8.2). Nerve roots traverse the epidural space before leaving the spinal canal taking with them a thin layer of membranes and a sleeve of dura that is continuous with the subarachnoid space. It is therefore possible to accidentally puncture intrathecally when lateral to the vertebra during stellate or paravertebral blocks.

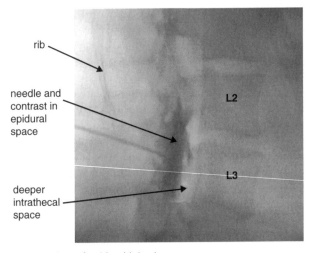

Fig. 8.2 Lateral view of epidural injection.

Anatomical issues in palliative care

There are anatomical issues that are specific to palliative care practice. Adequate investigation is necessary into the sources of pain before spinal drug administration is considered. MRI scans and other investigations that assess intrathecal disease or impending cord compression may be required.

- Positioning patients with overwhelming pain in order to perform spinal blocks may be very difficult.

- Ageing, disease, tumour, and degeneration of the spine narrow the exit foramina and may limit the lateral passage of injected solutions. This may mean that smaller volumes of epidural drugs than are usual are needed in these situations. It is important not to inject such large volumes that intraspinal pressure is increased.

- Any spinal injection in patients with increased intracranial pressure is hazardous since coning can occur.

- Vertebral metastases, spinal stenosis, loss of epidural fat in cachexia, and epidural invasion by tumour may complicate spinal drug administration and drug distribution.[5]

- ITDD may be compromised in those with tumour-related obstruction to CSF circulation.

- Intrathecal or epidural injection in those with impending cord compression can be hazardous, precipitating complete cord compression.

- Epidural injection should never be performed when there is resistance to flow of injectate since the pressure increase will displace CSF and transmit pressure intracranially.

- The epidural space is filled with fatty areolar tissue. Epidural veins are largely anterolateral and are valveless, so that they transmit intrathoracic and intra-abdominal pressures. Increased pressure from coughing, straining, tumour, or ascites may distend epidural veins and make accidental intravenous drug administration during spinal block more likely. Distension of these veins also reduces the volume of the epidural space so lower drug doses and volumes may be needed.

Indications for spinal drug delivery and test dosing

- Patients in whom systemic analgesia is effective but gives intolerable side-effects.

- Segmental pain or spasticity.

- Patients with indolent disease rather than those with a rapidly progressive, incident or changing patterns of pain.

- Patients who respond well to test dosing.

- Spinal drug delivery available from a centre with the experience and staffing to perform and support the techniques. The health care professionals involved must be skilled in implanting spinal systems, titrating spinal drugs and managing complications.

- Community staff available who know when to ask for specialist help for patients who are at home and using spinal systems.

It is important to find out whether the pain is sensitive to spinal drugs by administering one or more spinal test doses. This also allows the patient to experience the effects of spinal drugs before committing to long-term treatment. The choice of route and drugs for test dosing should mimic the technique under consideration for long-term treatment as closely as is practical. There is controversy about the relative merits of single bolus injections and indwelling temporary catheters for testing.

Advantages of single injection

- The procedure is simple

- The risk of infection is low

- The small needle size means that headache is unlikely.

Disadvantages of a single injection

- The effect is often brief so assessment can be difficult
- The patient gets less time to decide on the merits of the treatment
- If a single test injection is not effective, and there are no side-effects, then a further test may be needed with a higher dose or different combination of drugs.

The use of an epidural catheter to test for responsiveness to future intrathecal drug delivery may not be helpful. Some drugs do not cross the dura readily, so that the predictive value of epidural use is therefore uncertain. Dose equivalence is not clear which can lead to false negative testing. If an accidental dural puncture occurs using an epidural needle then a spinal headache is very likely. The use of a temporary external intrathecal catheter to predict response to ITDD is attractive because it allows various drugs and doses to be tried in a variety of situations over time. It has the disadvantages of requiring a larger needle to pass a catheter increasing the risk of headache. There may also be more risk of infection.

Contraindications to spinal drug delivery

Absolute contraindications

- Patient refusal
- Inadequate analgesia or intolerable side-effects from test dose
- Local or systemic infection
- Non-correctable co-aggulopathy
- Raised intracranial pressure
- Impending spinal cord compression
- Lack of support services in hospital, palliative care unit, or community.

Relative contraindications

- Current chemotherapy and neutropenia
- Spinal deformity or previous spinal surgery
- Neurological problems are not a contraindication to spinal drug use, but these must be carefully investigated and documented prior to the procedure
- Head pain is not well managed by ITDD (intra-cerebroventricular drug delivery may be an option).

Equipment for spinal drug delivery

Spinal drugs can be given as a single injection or a catheter can be introduced either epidurally or intrathecally for long-term drug administration. Needle and catheter design are important in determining the success and adverse effects of spinal analgesia.

Epidural techniques

The preferred needles for epidural injection are of a large diameter (14–18 G), usually have a side hole and are graduated in centimetres (cm) (such as a Tuohy needle) (Fig. 8.3). Catheters are marked in cm, so that it is possible to note how much catheter is placed in the epidural space. If a large epidural needle accidentally penetrates the dura, this causes a leak of CSF and a low-pressure spinal headache is very likely. The needles are designed to allow the passage of large gauge catheters that are used for short periods (usually less than a few days) in obstetric and surgical anaesthesia or intensive care. These simple catheters are unsuitable for long-term spinal infusion in palliative care practice. They are made of material that was not designed for prolonged use, they are not kink resistant and they are not radio-opaque. If prolonged spinal catheterization is planned then catheters designed for the purpose should be used, even though they are more expensive (Fig. 8.4).

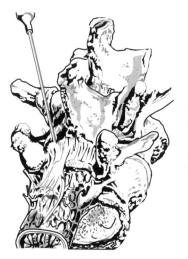 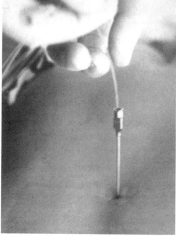

Fig. 8.3 Left: Anatomy of epidural injection. Right: Catheter insertion into the epidural space via a Tuohy needle.

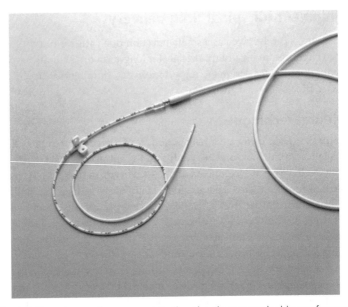

Fig. 8.4 Two-piece radio-opaque intrathecal catheters marked in cm for use with totally implanted systems.

Multiple side-holed radiopaque silicone rubber catheters are available. Some have a subcutaneous cuff that may improve fixation but this does not alter the infection rate. These are designed to be tunnelled subcutaneously and left in situ long term. Catheters are sometimes tunnelled to a subcutaneous port that is then accessed by a right-angled needle. These have no proven advantage over simpler systems and repeated needling to access the subcutaneous may increase the infection risk. Bacterial filters (0.22 μm) must be used at the patient and pump ends of the system—these must be changed as infrequently as possible such as every 1–2 months. Lines for spinal infusion should be a different colour to distinguish them from intravenous and feeding lines and reduce the risk of accidental injection or infusion of the wrong drugs.

Spinal techniques

Needles used for single, intrathecal puncture are of much smaller diameter (20–32 G) than epidural needles. There are various designs such as 45 degree bevel (Quinke), pencil point or side hole (such as a Sprotte). The likelihood of low-pressure spinal headache and of neural trauma are related to needle diameter and design. Micro-catheters were designed to go through small spinal needles for continuous intrathecal block in anaesthetic practice. These are unsuitable for palliative care practice because they readily become blocked. The silicone rubber catheters designed for epidural use are suitable for long-term subarachnoid placement. Fully implantable ITDD systems employ large needles (14–15 G) that have side holes and use silicone catheters (14–16 G); headache is therefore common after the procedure. Placement of intrathecal catheters is not associated with neurotoxicity assessed at post-mortem.

External portable pumps

These can be used to infuse spinal drugs in patients whose life expectancy is quite short (less than 3 months) or for those who may need larger volume infusions.[6] The pumps must be fit for the purpose with a large capacity (at least 250 ml) and the ability to give very low volume infusions with precision. The simple pumps commonly used for subcutaneous drug infusion in palliative care are not suitable for spinal drug delivery and must not be used because the chance of inaccurate infusion and accidental bolusing with these pumps is too great. It is vital that the system remains closed, that any access is as infrequent as possible and that when access is required it is performed with meticulous aseptic technique. Each unit must standardize the pumps used so that staff training and maintenance of equipment are as simple as possible. The need for education about the equipment used should never be underestimated and should be extended to community-based staff where appropriate. External spinal drug delivery will fail if attention to detail such as pump provision and staff education is neglected. Where these are not available the technique must not be used. Pumps must have adequate safety features:

- Simple programming
- Occlusion and volumetric alarms
- Lockable programming
- Anti-syphon systems
- Patient-controlled bolusing facilities can be useful for spinal drug administration, as long as care is taken with programming.[7]

Fully implantable ITDD pumps

Fully implantable ITDD pumps are most appropriate for patients with slowly progressive disease and whose life expectancy is measured in months. They are made of inert metals with some plastic components.

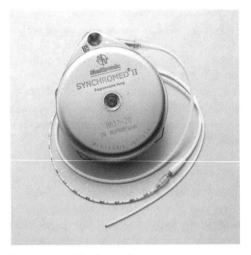

Fig. 8.5 Intrathecal pump: 40 ml capacity.

Such pumps are only practical for ITDD and cannot be used epidurally because the reservoir size is small. They may be gas driven and deliver a pre-set hourly drug dose. Alternatively, there may be an internal battery with a life of about 7 years with the infusion telemetrically controlled (Fig. 8.5). There may be a facility for patient-controlled intrathecal bolus dosing (Fig. 8.6). Pump volumes vary from 10–40 ml for the battery-powered pumps and 50 ml for the gas powered, constant rate pumps. The catheter is tunnelled to the anterior abdominal wall where the pump is implanted into a subcutaneous pocket so that the pump can be re-filled percutaneously. Occasionally patients may be allergic to catheter or pump components; this may present with features similar to infection and often necessitates removal of the system. However, in most cases, once the immediate discomfort has resolved, implantable pumps are much easier for the patient to manage. The main inconvenience is the need to return to a medical environment for pump refills (Fig. 8.7).

Techniques for spinal drug administration

Spinal drug delivery is an invasive procedure that must be performed in an environment where full sterility can be maintained. Resuscitation facilities and trained assistants are mandatory. The use of fluoroscopy to guide catheter placement is important, as spinal drug delivery can be complicated for anatomical reasons in palliative care practice.

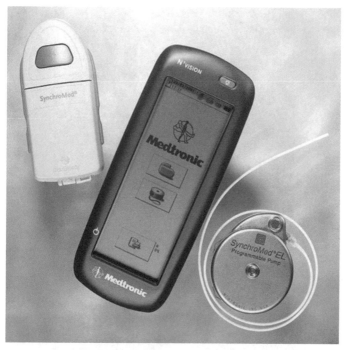

Fig. 8.6 Totally implantable intrathecal drug delivery system. Left to right: Personal programmer, a hand-held device that allows the patient to give a bolus intrathecally from the pump within preset parameters of dose and lockout time. Pump programmer that allows the therapist to set the intrathecal infusion parameters and check the volumes remaining in the pump at refill. Intrathecal pump with central filling port that takes a 22 G needle and meshed side access port that takes a 25 G needle and one-piece catheter.

Simple single injection

Single injections can be performed either epidurally or intrathecally with the patient awake, as long as they can be made comfortable for the procedure either sitting, leaning forward, or curled in the lateral position. The risk of spinal cord or neural trauma is reduced if verbal contact is maintained with the patient. If anxiety or pain prevents optimal positioning, then analgesia and sedation should be carefully administered.

External spinal systems

External spinal systems may be placed under local anaesthesia, but sometimes positioning is too painful and sedation or general anaesthesia is

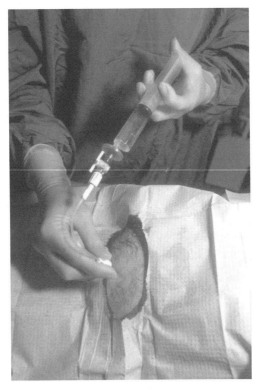

Fig. 8.7 Percutaneous refilling of fully implanted intrathecal drug delivery system; full asepsis is needed.

needed. The catheter should be inserted with the tip as near as possible to the dermatome of pain origin but high enough to deal with any predicted disease progression. Catheters may be externalized through the skin at the puncture site but it is better to tunnel them subcutaneously well away from the spine. If a superficial infection does occur, then it is distant from the spinal canal.

Fully implantable ITDD systems

Fully implantable systems are usually implanted under general anaesthesia. The intrathecal component may be difficult to place and the pump pocket is quite large so dissection under local anaesthesia can be distressing.

Choice of route and spinal system

Intrathecal delivery

Drugs do not have to pass the physical barrier of the dura to get to their site of action and so can be used in lower doses (usually 10–20% of the epidural dose). This is an important advantage when compared to the frequency of syringe driver or pump refills necessary to maintain analgesia with an external epidural system. However, fears about infection have caused some reluctance to use the intrathecal route.

Epidural delivery

Large-volume epidural injections or infusions may precipitate spinal cord compression. Epidural invasion by tumour and spinal stenosis are very common in patients who present for spinal drug delivery. These problems can compromise epidural drug administration. Changes in the amount of epidural fat in those with cancer can also influence drug delivery.

General complications

In the first 20 days after implant there are more problems with the intrathecal (25%) than the epidural (8%) route. However, the expected complication of headache from CSF leak is the main problem after intrathecal catheterization within the first 20 days and this can be managed with simple analgesia and intravenous fluid replacement if necessary. Thereafter the complication rate for epidural drug administration rises to 55% and intrathecal falls to 5%.[8]

Fibrosis

During the first 20 days, catheters placed in the epidural space are more likely to become blocked by fibrosis than intrathecal catheters; this may lead to loss of analgesia and local pain during epidural injection or infusion. However, there have been reports of symptomatic intrathecal granulomas with long-term intrathecal catheters. This may be related to the use of multiple drugs or high doses of morphine and is usually more of an issue in patients with chronic, non-cancer related pain.

Infection

Close monitoring and a high index of suspicion are needed in all patients with spinal systems. A single dose of a broad-spectrum antibiotic should be given at the time of catheter insertion—advice from a microbiologist with knowledge of local infection control policies may be useful when choosing suitable antibiotics. The prophylactic use of antibiotics after catheter placement does not reduce the infection risk. Local infections around the catheter, epidural abscess, and meningitis are serious risks; pathogens are usually skin flora. The catheter hub is the commonest site for entry of infection. One risk factor for infection is a time of more than 100 minutes taken to place the catheter. This may be because of patient factors or a general reflection of the unit's experience with spinal drug delivery. These are not techniques for the occasional user.

Epidural catheters have a high rate of infection and technical complications. In a study of 91 patients with 137 epidural catheters over a period of 4326 catheter-days, 43% had technical complications and 12 patients had deep infections (11 with epidural abscess); this is unacceptable.[9] There is no evidence that externalized, tunnelled intrathecal catheters have a higher infection rate than epidural catheters. Infection risk is not a valid reason to restrict external catheters to patients within the last few weeks of life. Reported infection rates vary between 1 per 150 to 1 per 7250 catheter-days. In a study of 200 adults with external intrathecal catheters treated for 1–575 days, where there were defined protocols for catheter care, 93% had perfect function of the system. Infection was recorded as follows: catheter site entry 0.5%, catheter track 0%, epidural abscess 0%, meningitis 0.5%, systemic infection 0%. This gave an infection rate of 1 per 7242 treatment-days.[3] Sub-clinical occult infection may be commoner than realized with one study showing that about 20% cultures from cassettes, syringes, and filters were colonized without clinical evidence of infection.[10] The infection rate can be kept low with careful attention to asepsis. Sound protocols for the care of patients having spinal drugs are very important.

Overall it has been clear since the early 1990s that ITDD from either external or totally internal systems provides better pain control and fewer complications than epidural drug administration.[11, 12] ITDD has:

- Lower incidence of catheter occlusion
- Lower malfunction rate
- Lower dose requirement
- Fewer side-effects
- Better pain control
- No increased risk of infection.

Choice of drugs

Many different drugs have been administered spinally. It has been suggested that opioids should initially be used alone and that other drugs should only be added if analgesia is inadequate.[13] However, multi-modal analgesia may allow the use of lower doses of individual drugs and limit side-effects. Spinal toxicity of drugs and their preservatives must be considered; morphine (with and without preservative), hydromorphone, bupivacaine, clonidine, and baclofen are not neurotoxic. Stability of drugs in CSF over time and at different temperatures is important when choosing drugs. Bupivacaine, morphine, hydromorphone, clonidine, and baclofen have all been shown to be stable at room and body temperature for at least 3 months so their long-term stability when used in spinal systems is not a problem.[14–16]

Opioids

There are few randomized, controlled trials of long-term spinal opioids and a lack of consensus about the appropriate method of converting systemic to spinal drug doses. It is usual to start with a low dose of spinal opioid in addition to 50% of the usual systemic opioid dose. The spinal dose is then titrated up whilst the systemic dose is reduced; in this way symptoms of withdrawal can be prevented.

Lipid solubility is an important consideration when choosing an opioid. Water-soluble drugs have a greater relative potency than those that are more lipid soluble when given spinally (Table 8.1). All spinal opioids can cause respiratory depression, sedation, confusion, emesis, constipation, retention of urine, and itching.

Morphine is the most *water soluble* (hydrophilic) opioid used spinally. Intrathecal morphine is about ten times as potent as the same dose given epidurally and that is in turn ten times more potent than systemic morphine. Intrathecal morphine has a slower onset and longer duration of action than other more lipid-soluble drugs that are carried away in the blood. It dissolves readily in the CSF and is therefore more likely to spread rostrally causing respiratory depression. However, internationally most experience with spinal drug delivery has been accumulated with morphine.

Table 8.1 Characteristics of drugs administered spinally by relative water and lipid solubility

	High lipid solubility	High water solubility
Relative potency, spinal vs. systemic	Low	High
Rostral spread in CSF	Low	High
Volume of distribution following spinal infusion	High	Low

Diamorphine is available in the UK; it is convenient for spinal use because it can be mixed as a very concentrated solution reducing the need for frequent syringe driver or pump refills. It is a prodrug of morphine but is highly *lipid soluble*. It may enter the nerve roots and spinal cord more readily than morphine. There is limited data on its stability. Diamorphine is not now recommended for fully implantable ITDD systems as pump failure has been reported when very concentrated solutions are used.

Hydromorphone is about five times as potent as morphine. It is lipid soluble and available in powder form that can be useful if concentrated solutions are needed.

There is limited data on the use of spinal *methadone*; the *N*-methyl-D-aspartate (NMDA) receptor activity (see below) of the d-isomer may not be clinically significant.

The use of spinal *fentanyl* has been widely studied. It is a potent, *lipid-soluble* opioid that is rapidly cleared when given epidurally and results in significant plasma concentrations that may contribute to analgesia. *Sufentanil* is available in some countries. It is a potent, *lipid-soluble* opioid similar to fentanyl. It leaves the intrathecal compartment and enters the cord, epidural space, and blood vessels. Neurotoxicity has been suggested in animal studies of high sufentanil doses but there are no clinical studies that support this.

Local anaesthetics

There is most experience with the use of spinal local anaesthetics with ample data about efficacy, dose, side-effects, and stability. *Bupivacaine* is most commonly used. *Ropivacaine* may be less cardiotoxic, but in a concentration of 0.5% it has not been shown to be superior to bupivacaine in terms of neural blockade.[17] *Levobupivacaine* is also less cardiotoxic than bupivacaine. The use of local anaesthetics with opioids may reduce opioid tolerance. It has been suggested that about 90% patients with pain refractory to epidural opioids alone can regain analgesia when opioid is combined with bupivacaine. The dose of intrathecal bupivacaine must be kept below 30–60 mg (equivalent to 6–12 ml of 0.5%) daily to minimize adverse effects such as numbness and motor block;[18] the total daily dose is more important than the concentration. CNS or systemic toxicity is rare, even with plasma concentrations of more than 10 μg/ml. Injection of a large dose of local anaesthetic may produce a 'total spinal' (see below). Care must be taken that local anaesthetic infusions are not assumed to be the cause of neurological symptoms and signs such as increasing numbness or motor block that may signal spinal cord compression. In patients with extensive disease the use of local anaesthetics may be the only option. In some cases numbness has to be the accepted price of good analgesia. On occasions the provision of sensory block is needed—particularly in the last few days of life. It is important to realize that despite good analgesia from this the patient may need their distress managing pharmacologically or by other methods.

Clonidine

Spinal clonidine is widely used in acute pain. Case series and reports show that clonidine can be a useful adjunct to spinal opioids, especially in those with neuropathic pain, but there is little data on long-term use. It has a synergistic affect with opioids. As an α-2 adrenoceptor agonist it may cause sedation, bradycardia, and hypotension. Usual starting doses are 50–75 µg/day epidurally or 10–20 µg/day intrathecally.

Ketamine

Glutamate is the most important excitatory transmitter in the nervous system exerting some of its effect via the NMDA receptor. Ketamine is an NMDA antagonist that is analgesic when given to animals by the spinal route. A preservative-free formulation is available but it can be difficult to obtain. There is some animal evidence that the preservatives used in the injectable formulation are not neurotoxic. Ketamine has been used spinally for acute and chronic pain. Some of its analgesic effect after spinal delivery may be related to systemic absorption. It has side-effects such as sedation and may cause subtle or florid mood changes. On available evidence it cannot be recommended for routine use.

Baclofen

Intrathecal administration of baclofen (a gamma-aminobutyric acid-B receptor blocker) is standard therapy for spasticity. The dose can vary from 25–1200 µg/day. There has been animal and preliminary clinical work suggesting that it may have analgesic efficacy and it may be considered in some refractory pain problems. Side-effects include muscle weakness and sedation so very low doses should be used initially. Standard intrathecal test doses in adult patients with spasticity range from 25–75 µg; however, in those with normal muscles the test dose may need to be reduced. Care must be taken to avoid acute baclofen withdrawal as this may lead to serious side-effects e.g. fits or psychosis.

Other drugs

Octreotide, midazolam, neostigmine, droperidol, aspirin, non-steroidal anti-inflammatory drugs, and ziconotide (a calcium channel blocking toxin) have all been used spinally in animals and man with variable results. There is not enough clinical data to support their routine use.

Complications and management

Total spinal

Injection of a large dose of local anaesthetic intrathecally, especially as a bolus may result in a 'total spinal'. In an adult 5–6 ml of 0.5% bupivacaine produces a very high block. The effects of the anaesthetic on the brain stem lead to cardio-respiratory collapse that requires aggressive resuscitation including tracheal intubation, ventilation, fluids, and drugs.

Spinal headache

Low-pressure spinal headache can occur after any intrathecal puncture— however, the incidence is related to needle size and design. Headache is very likely after accidental dural puncture with a large epidural needle or during placement of an intrathecal catheter and is more likely in young females. It is less common when there is spinal stenosis. The headache is severe, often occipital, worsened by sitting or standing and lying flat relieves it. It may be accompanied by emesis and photo/phonophobia. Rarely, other localizing signs such as sixth nerve palsy occur but in a palliative care setting this should prompt further investigation. It should be treated using standard analgesics. It is often less of a problem in palliative care because patients are already receiving a variety of analgesics. Various treatments have been described such as aggressive rehydration, lying prone, abdominal binders, epidural saline infusion, caffeine, and sumatriptan. None of these has proven efficacy. The definitive management is epidural blood patch. This involves placement of 20–30 ml autologous blood into the epidural space above or below the puncture site. The risks and benefits of this treatment need to be assessed in each case, as low-pressure headache is usually a self-limiting problem that usually settles within 7–10 days.

Bleeding

Prior to spinal drug delivery, co-aggulation status should be normal and anti-platelet drugs should be stopped for 10 days since bleeding into the epidural space may produce spinal compression (see below). Surgical bleeding can occur during or after ITDD implant; pump pocket haematoma must be evacuated promptly as this poses an infection risk.

Infection

Patients having spinal drugs must be carefully monitored for symptoms and signs of infection—those with indwelling systems are at greatest risk. Regular temperature monitoring, wound checks, and measurement of white blood count are important in the immediate postoperative period. If there is a suspicion of infection then a full infection screen and blood cultures are mandatory. Intercurrent infections such as chest or urinary tract infections may lead to a bacteraemia and subsequent catheter infection necessitating prompt assessment and treatment in patients with ITDD systems. Superficial skin infection around the exit site of a tunneled external catheter may be managed by appropriate intravenous antibiotic therapy. The patient must be observed for any signs of progression of infection that can happen alarmingly rapidly. If the problem does not resolve quickly then the system should be removed. Pump pocket infections are more serious. There have been reports that these can be managed using antibiotics but this is a risky strategy and should be abandoned early if unsuccessful. The patient must be observed for signs of epidural abscess or meningitis.

Epidural abscess presents with the triad of:

- Back pain
- Fever
- Variable neurological signs and symptoms.

MRI scanning should be performed early as neurological changes often occur late or may be absent until the situation has progressed beyond the stage of recovery.

Meningitis may present in a very insidious manner and classical signs such as neck stiffness or photophobia may be masked by the analgesics.

If there are any signs of spinal infection, then it is essential that the whole system be removed and that the infection is managed aggressively. Advice may be needed from radiology, microbiology, and surgical colleagues when managing patients with infection.

Local pain

Patients may experience pain on bolus injection or infusion through epidural catheters. This is usually due to catheter tip fibrosis and often necessitates the removal of the system.

Dose escalation

Disease progression rather than tolerance is usually the major factor behind dose escalation. There is no evidence that this is related to duration of drug administration. In this situation spinal opioid switching or the use of alternative or additional intrathecal drugs may be considered.

Drug withdrawal

Acute pain and drug withdrawal reactions can occur if intrathecal drug delivery is abruptly terminated for any reason. This should be managed with appropriate parenteral drugs; smaller doses than expected may be needed so titration should be done with care and adequate monitoring. The patient and their carers must know how to obtain immediate advice in this urgent situation. It is important to remain vigilant for other causes of symptoms and signs, and not to make the assumption that every problem is related to spinal drugs.

Drug side-effects

All intrathecal drugs produce side-effects that should be monitored and managed. *Sedation, confusion,* or *hypotension* may necessitate dose changes or drug switching. *Emesis* is usually temporary and should be managed using standard therapy; if it persists then drug switching may be needed.

Itch from opioids may be treated with drugs such as ondansetron.

Sensory or motor blockade with local anaesthetics should be adequately investigated. This may require reduction in the local anaesthetic dose that is not always possible without loss of analgesia.

Long-term intrathecal opioid use has *endocrine and immune effects* although the significance of these is not clear.

Altered *sexual function* may occur that may respond to hormonal treatment.

Spinal cord and nerve injury

It is possible to cause trauma to neural tissues during spinal drug administration. The best way to minimize the risk is to perform injections and catheter insertions with the patient awake. In this way the operator can be alerted by complaints of paraesthesia or pain. However, it is not always desirable or feasible for patients to be awake during procedures and the risks have to be balanced against the benefits for each case. Patients must be informed about such risks.

Spinal cord or cauda equina compression

If a patient develops new neurological symptoms and signs during spinal drug delivery then spinal cord or cauda equina compression should be suspected.[19] Haematoma or epidural abscess may cause compression. Back pain, pyrexia and leukocytosis can occur early. Autonomic, sensory, and motor problems come later. Sterile granulomas may also occur at the catheter tip during spinal drug delivery.[20, 21] This may be related to the position of the catheter being ventral within the spine where there is slow flow of CSF. It may also be related to high drug concentrations. Early MRI scanning and support from a neuro-radiologist is important if spinal compression is suspected. It is often possible to MRI scan patients with ITDD systems in situ. The manufacturers advice should be sought and the pump must be turned off.

Terminal Care

As the patient approaches the end of life the pain may change in character or distribution. The small pump reservoir may mean that, at this stage, an alternative method of analgesia must be used. It is important not to rely on the pump to solve a pain problem that it was never intended to manage and to be ready to use other methods as an adjunct or even an alternative.

Conclusions

A multi-disciplinary approach is crucial for successful patient selection and management when considering spinal drugs. Patients, families, and staff need to understand the goals and limitations of spinal drug delivery. All staff caring for the patient in hospital, hospice, or community must be trained in the on-going management of spinal infusions. Adverse effects must be diagnosed and treated quickly. Regular assessment of patients is important, especially with regard to infection or impending neurological problems. Spinal drug delivery is highly effective in a selected group of patients with difficult to control malignant pain.[22, 23]

Further reading

Brown DL (1999). *Atlas of regional anesthesia*, 2nd edn. W B Saunders Company, Philadelphia, PA.

Hahn MB, McQuillan PM, and Sheplock GJ (1996). *Regional anaesthesia: an atlas of anatomy and techniques*. Mosby, St Louis, MO.

Raj PP, Lou L, Erdine S, *et al.* (2003). *Radiographic imaging for regional anaesthesia and pain management*. Churchill Livingstone, Edinburgh.

References

1. Staats P (1999). Neuraxial infusion for pain control: When, why, and what to do after the implant. *Oncology* **13**:58–62.

2. Buchheit T and Rauck R (1999). Subarachnoid techniques for cancer pain therapy: when, why and how? *Curr Rev Pain* **3**:198–205.

3. Nitescu P, Sjoberg M, Applegren L, *et al.* (1995). Complications of intrathecal opioids and bupivacaine in the treatment of 'refractory' cancer pain. *Clin J Pain* **11**:45–62.

4. Smith TJ, Staats PS, Deer T, *et al.* (2002). Randomized clinical trial of an implantable drug delivery system compared with comprehensive medical management for refractory cancer pain: impact on pain, drug-related toxicity and survival. *J Clin Oncol* **20**:4040–9.

5. Appelgren L, Nordborg C, Sjoberg M, *et al.* (1997). Spinal epidural metastasis: implications for spinal analgesia to treat 'refractory' cancer pain. *J Pain Symptom Manage* **13**:25–42.

6. Hassenbusch SJ, Paice JA, Patt RB, *et al.* (1997). Clinical realities and economic considerations: economics of intrathecal therapy. *J Pain Symptom Manage* **14**(Suppl 3):S36–48.

7. Tumber PS and Fitzgibbon DR (1998). The control of severe cancer pain by continuous intrathecal and patient controlled intrathecal analgesia with morphine, bupivacaine and clonidine. *Pain* **78**:217–20.

8. Crul BJ and Delhaas EM (1991). Technical complications during long-term subarachnoid or epidural administration of morphine in terminally ill cancer patients: a review of 140 cases. *Reg Anesth* **16**:209–13.

9. Smitt PS, Tsafka A, Teng-ran de Zande F, *et al.* (1998). Outcome and complications of epidural analgesia in patients with chronic cancer pain. *Cancer* **83**:2015–22.

10. Nitescu P, Hultman E, Applegren L, *et al.* (1992). Bacteriology, drug stability and exchange of percutaneous delivery systems and antibacterial filters in long-term intrathecal infusion of opioid drugs and bupivacaine in 'refractory' pain. *Clin J Pain* **8**:324–37.

11. Nitescu P, Applegren L, Linder LE, *et al.* (1990). Epidural versus intrathecal morphine-bupivacaine: assessment of consecutive treatments in advanced cancer pain. *J Pain Symptom Manage* **5**:18–26.

12. Dahm P, Nitescu P, Appelgren L, *et al.* (1998). Efficacy and technical complications of long-term continuous intraspinal infusions of opioid and/or bupivacaine in refractory non-malignant pain: a comparison between the epidural and the intrathecal approach with externalised or implanted catheters and infusion pumps. *Clin J Pain* **14**:4–16.

13. Bennett G, Burchiel K, Buchser E, *et al.* (2000). Clinical guidelines for intraspinal infusion: Report of an expert panel. *J Pain Symptom Manage* **20**:S37–43.

14. Hildebrand KR, Elsberry DD, and Deer TR (2001). Stability, compatibility, and safety of intrathecal bupivacaine administered chronically via an implantable delivery system. *Clin J Pain* **17**:239–44.

15. Hildebrand KR, Elsberry DD, and Hassenbusch SJ (2003). Stability and compatibility of morphine-clonidine admixtures in an implantable infusion system. *J Pain Symptom Manage* **25**:464–71.

16. Hildebrand KR, Elsberry DD, and Anderson VC (2001). Stability and compatibility of hydromorphone hydrochloride in an implantable infusion system. *J Pain Symptom Manage* **22**:1042–7.

17. Dahm P, Lundborg C, Janson M, *et al.* (2000). Comparison of 0.5% intrathecal bupivacaine with 0.5% intrathecal ropivacaine in the treatment of refractory cancer and non-cancer pain conditions: results from a prospective, crossover, double-blind, randomised study. *Reg Anesth Pain Med* **25**:480–7.

18. Mercadante S (1999). Problems of long-term spinal opioid treatment in advanced cancer patients. *Pain* **79**:1–13.

19. Van Dongen RT, van EE, and Crul BJ (1997). Neurological impairment during long-term intrathecal infusion of bupivacaine in cancer patients: a sign of spinal cord compression. *Pain* **69**:205–9.

20. McMillan MR, Doud T, and Nugent W (2003). Catheter-associated masses in patients receiving intrathecal analgesic therapy. *Anesth Analg* **96**:186–90.

21. Coffey RJ and Burchiel K (2002). Inflammatory mass lesions associated with intrathecal drug infusion catheters: report and observations on 41 patients. *Neurosurgery* **50**:78–86.

22. Bennett G, Serafini M, Burchiel K, *et al.* (2000). Evidence-based reviews of the literature on intrathecal delivery of pain medication. *J Pain Symptom Manage* **20**:S12–36.

23. Bennett G, Deer T, Du Pen S, *et al.* (2000). Future directions in the management of pain by intraspinal drug delivery. *J Pain Symptom Manage* **20**:S44–50.

9

Electrical stimulation techniques

Sensory stimulation and modulation have been used to provide analgesia in various forms for many centuries. Established methods include counter irritation, scarification, cauterization, cupping, and acupuncture. More recently transcutaneous nerve stimulation (TENS) and spinal cord stimulation (SCS) have been developed, based on the gate theory of pain modulation (Fig. 9.1).

Acupuncture

Acupuncture has become standard therapy in many pain and palliative care services, in the management of pain and other symptoms such as emesis and dyspnoea. Acupuncture has been used for a wide variety of chronic pain problems, with variable success[1] (Fig. 9.2). There is little evidence from systematic reviews concerning the efficacy of acupuncture for pain management.[2] However, there are problems inherent in designing good acupuncture trials that should be considered when interpreting research findings.[3] Much work remains to be done on the choice of optimal stimulation for selected pain problems in cancer patients.[4]

Techniques

The usual approach is based on a combination of segmental point selection, trigger point therapy, and the use of some traditional Chinese points. There are various types of stimulation that can be used for acupuncture, such as acupressure, manual needling, electrical stimulation, or laser stimulation. Various frequencies and intensities of stimulation have differing effects on the release of neurotransmitters. Sometimes acupuncture is used in specific areas, as in auricular treatment. Some patients are more sensitive to acupuncture than others, and can be described as strong reactors.

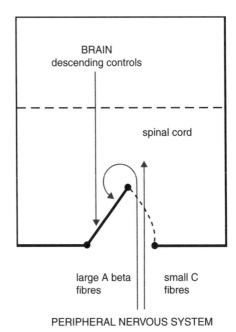

BRAIN
descending controls

spinal cord

large A beta
fibres

small C
fibres

PERIPHERAL NERVOUS SYSTEM

Fig. 9.1 Gating of pain. Stimulation of peripheral large A beta fibres closes the 'gate' at spinal level and inhibits upward transmission of pain via A delta and C fibres. There is also descending gating from the brain that inhibits pain transmission.

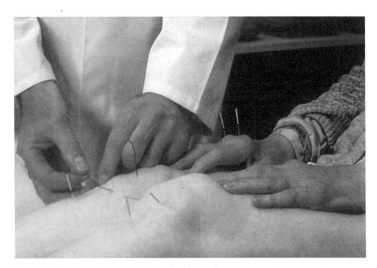

Fig. 9.2 Acupuncture treatment of arthritic knees.

Trigger point therapy is used for a wide variety of musculoskeletal and visceral disorders. A segmental approach to treatment relevant to the affected dermatomes, myotomes, and sclerotomes can be used. Strong traditional analgesic points such as large intestine 4 on the dorsum of the hand and liver and 3 on the foot are often helpful.

Contraindications

- Gross clotting dysfunction
- Local infection
- Care in diabetics or those at risk of endocarditis
- Pregnancy in case of inducing a miscarriage
- Needles should not be inserted directly into superficial sites of tumour
- Needles should not be used in the limbs of patients with moderate to severe lymphoedema (contralateral needling can be used)
- Electroacupuncture should not be used in those who have a pacemaker
- Needling should not be performed around the area of an unstable spine, this may remove protective muscle spasm.

Adverse effects

Acupuncture has few side-effects, when appropriately trained and experienced staff perform it carefully.[5] A sound knowledge of anatomy, and the use of sterile disposable needles are important for safe treatment. It is vital that the acupuncturist has adequate training and skills. Specific complications include:

- Minor side-effects (such as bleeding, bruising, post needling pain, sedation and mood change)
- Serious adverse effects (such as pneumothorax, haemothorax, hepatitis, endocarditis, pericarditis, septicaemia, cardiac tamponade, compartment syndrome, cardiovascular or neural trauma, retained needles, burns from moxibustion, and death).

Transcutaneous electrical nerve stimulation (TENS)

Mode of action

In 1967 Wall and Sweet showed that high-frequency (50–100 Hz) percutaneous electrical nerve stimulation relieved chronic neuropathic pain.[6] Transcutaneous electrical nerve stimulation was then used to try to select patients for spinal cord stimulation (SCS).[7] It was shown that TENS was an effective therapy in its own right, but it did not predict the response to SCS. More recent developments of TENS have involved the use of different patterns of electrical stimulation such as pulsed ('burst'), modulation (ramped), random and complex waveforms that are all designed to try to improve the efficacy of TENS. It has been proposed that the effect of low frequency TENS is mediated via pro-enkephalin derived peptides acting on μ receptors, and that high-frequency stimulation releases dynorphinergic-like substances with the analgesic effects mediated via κ opioid receptors. Low-frequency stimulation produces an almost fourfold increase in metenkephalin measured in the lumbar spinal fluid, whereas high-frequency stimulation resulted in a 49% increase in dynorphin. On this basis, several other studies have chosen to use the mixed frequency 'dense-and-disperse' mode of stimulation. The duration and timing of stimulations is another variable between studies. Intermittent stimulation for short intervals of around 30 minutes may be more effective than prolonged or continuous stimulation as the development of tolerance may reduce effectiveness. It takes about 30 minutes for analgesia to develop and plateau, and around 45 minutes for pain thresholds to return to baseline values following cessation of stimulation.

There has been increasing interest from pain practitioners and cardiologists in the role of TENS in the management of angina, despite a lack of evidence based on randomized controlled trials. The evidence from clinical experience and case reports is encouraging, and studies investigating the physiological basis of observed clinical effects provide a rationale for its use. Clinicians have used TENS in the management of patients with severe refractory angina not responding satisfactorily to medical or surgical treatment, on patients waiting for surgery and in those intolerant of nitrates. It has been shown that treatment with TENS can both significantly improve tolerance to pacing and myocardial lactate metabolism. This effect has not been found to be naloxone reversible and so is not a beta-endorphin mediated effect. It may be related to the delta or kappa receptor agonists, met-enkephalin, or dynorphin. Other studies suggest that a reduction in sympathetic tone is important and that TENS has its effect by reducing myocardial oxygen consumption.

Evidence of effectiveness

As with medication, there is a placebo response to TENS and this contributes to the initial, but transient analgesic effect seen with some patients. Meta-analyses of randomized, controlled trials of TENS produced mixed conclusions.[8, 9] The quality of the trials was variable. None of the TENS trials were blinded, as this is much more difficult than blinding in drug studies. Outcome measures should be about pain intensity or pain relief, and not indirect measures such as the need to use other analgesic interventions or a reduction of analgesic consumption. The dose of TENS used must be adequate. The conclusion was that the use of TENS in chronic pain might be justified, although this remains to be proven.

Equipment

TENS equipment should have the following features[10] (Fig. 9.3):

- Compact, lightweight, robust, and attachable to a belt or pocket
- On and off, amplitude and frequency controls of convenient size and shape, easily accessible and adjustable
- Controls protected from accidental knocking or disturbance
- Variable pulse patterns available
- Low battery drain
- Lightweight, flexible leads connecting to standard electrodes.
- Electrode pads should be disposable and self adhesive and available in a variety of sizes
- Hypoallergenic electrode pads should be available
- Clear patient information and instruction manual.

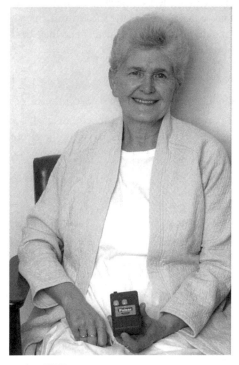

Fig. 9.3 Patient using TENS.

It is important for staff training and equipment maintenance that departments standardize on a maximum of two types of stimulator that have been found by patients, nurses, and medical staff to be effective and reliable.

Techniques

When initiating TENS therapy it is important to establish that the electrode positions employed are optimum. This may take a considerable amount of time and patience on the part of both patient and therapist. Success with TENS depends on giving patients clear instructions and ongoing support with treatment. Standard electrode positions based on a dermatomal or myotomal pain pattern have been suggested. The TENS sensation should cover the painful area. The sensation produced should be 'strong but comfortable', and not just tolerable. Muscle spasm should not occur when using conventional or pulsed TENS. In acupuncture-like TENS the stimulus is adjusted to a strength that evokes muscle twitching. The patient should be encouraged to alter the sites of electrode application, and to try a variety of electrode configurations; to treat large areas of pain, multiple electrodes may be needed. It is often useful initially to place electrodes over the painful site and stimulate. If this is not effective, then the electrodes should be placed over the next largest nerve that innervates the affected area. Initially patients using TENS therapy should be reviewed frequently and their treatment adjusted according to response.[11, 12]

Contraindications

- Electrodes should not be applied to inflamed, infected, or unhealthy skin
- The anterior part of the neck must not be stimulated to avoid the possibility of stimulating the nerves of the larynx or the carotid sinus
- Pregnancy
- Cardiac pacemaker.

Adverse effects

Ensuring that the area where electrodes are applied is kept dry, clean, and free from grease can minimize complications; electrical resistance between the electrode and skin is thus kept low and evenly distributed. Serious complications due to TENS therapy are rare and include:

- Equipment failure due to faulty leads, stimulator, battery or charger
- Skin irritation
- Skin burn
- Allergy to the electrodes.

Spinal cord stimulation (SCS)

Inspired by the gate control theory and animal studies, Shealy implanted a spinal cord stimulator into a man with pain from a chest wall cancer.[13] He obtained relief, with no impairment of vibration, position, touch, or pinprick sensations, although deep pain sensation was felt as touch. Shealy reported five further patients with various pathologies including cancer. Good results were obtained in spite of four patients having perineal pain, normally a difficult area to target. Several early series included small numbers of patients with cancer-related pain and showed variable results. It is likely that only neuropathic cancer pain responds to SCS. However, as techniques and equipment improve it is likely that SCS will be applicable to more pain conditions.[14]

Technique

An electrode is placed in the epidural space under local anaesthetic (Fig. 9.4); a pulse generator is placed in the abdomen to provide the stimulating current. During electrode placement, the patient needs to tell the operator

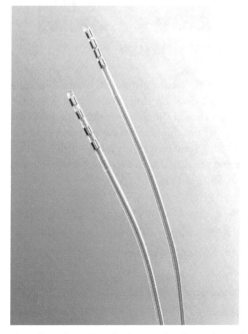

Fig. 9.4 Examples of quadrapolar spinal cord stimulator electrodes.

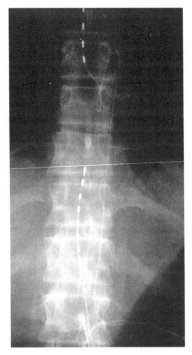

Fig. 9.5 Dual spinal cord stimulator electrodes in situ.

whether the correct electrode position has been achieved, so that paraesthesiae are produced over the whole area of pain. The electrode position and configuration chosen should cover the widest dermatomal area, so that if the pain spreads, the stimulation pattern may be altered to cope with this (Fig. 9.5). A second electrode can be introduced to increase stimulation. Some areas remain difficult to target selectively such as the lower back, perineum, and genitalia.

Indications
- Pain following back surgery
- Complex regional pain syndrome
- Nerve plexus pain
- Peripheral nerve pain
- Cauda equina pain
- Amputation and stump pain

- Refractory angina
- Peripheral vascular pain.

Contraindications

- Axial pain such as in the rectum, vagina, perineum
- Nociceptive pain
- Incident pain
- Widespread malignancy
- Diffuse pain
- Life expectancy less than 3 months.

Complications

- Infection and wound problems
- Electrode migration, dislodgement, lead fracture, and current leakage.

Further reading

Baldry PE (1993). *Acupuncture, trigger points and musculo-skeletal pain*, 2nd edn. Churchill Livingstone, Edinburgh.

Filshie J and White A (1998). *Medical acupuncture: a western scientific approach*. Churchill Livingstone, Edinburgh.

Rushton DN (2002). Electrical stimulation in the treatment of pain. *Disabil Rehabil* **24**, 407–15.

References

1. Hester J (1998). Acupuncture in the pain clinic. In: Filshie J and White A (ed.), *Medical acupuncture: a western scientific approach*, pp. 319–40. Churchill Livingstone, Edinburgh.

2. Ernst E and White AR (1998). Acupuncture for back pain: a meta-analysis of randomized controlled trials. *Arch Int Med* **158**:2235–41.

3. Hammerschlag R (1998). Methodological and ethical issues in clinical trials of acupuncture. *J Alt Comp Med* **4**:159–71.

4. Filshie J (1990). Acupuncture for malignant pain. *acup Med* **8**:38–9.

5. Rampes H and James R (1995). Complications of acupuncture. *Acup Medicine* **13**:26–33.

6. Wall PD and Sweet W (1967). Temporary abolition of pain in man. *Science* **155**: 108–9.

7. Long DM (1973). Electrical stimulation for relief of pain from chronic nerve injury. *J Neurosurg* **39**:718–22.

8. McQuay H and Moore A (1998). Transcutaneous electrical nerve stimulation (TENS) in chronic pain. In: *An evidence-based resource for pain relief*, pp. 207–11. Oxford University Press, Oxford.

9. Carroll D, Moore RA, McQuay HJ, *et al.* (2001). Transcutaneous electrical nerve stimulation (TENS) for chronic pain. *Cochrane Database Syst Rev* **3**:CD003222.

10. Reeve J, Menon D, and Corabian P (1996). Transcutaneous electrical nerve stimulation (TENS): a technology assessment. *International Journal of Technology Assessment in Health Care* **12**:299–324.

11. Johnson MI, Ashton CH, and Thompson JW (1991). An in-depth study of long-term users of transcutaneous electrical nerve stimulators (TENS). Implications for clinical use of TENS. *Pain* **44**:221–9.

12. Johnson MI, Ashton CH, and Thompson JW (1993). A prospective investigation into factors related to patient response to transcutaneous electrical nerve stimulation (TENS)—the importance of cortical responsivity. *Eur J Pain* **14**:1–9.

13. Shealy CN, Mortimer JT, and Reswick JB (1967) Electrical inhibition of pain by stimulation of the dorsal column: preliminary clinical reports. *Anesth Analg* **46**:488–91.

14. Barolat G and Sharan A (2000). Future trends in spinal cord stimulation. *Neurol Res* **22**:279–84.

10

Ethical issues

The principles behind the ethics of medical practice in palliative care are no different from those of other areas of medicine. This is important to remember when the complexity of some situations makes decision-making difficult. Before ethical considerations can be applied to particular areas of practice, an understanding of ethical concepts/moral philosophy is necessary.

The application of moral philosophy/ethics to medical practice helps to develop an understanding of how and why certain decisions may be made and to build a framework for careful thought when decisions are finely balanced. Personal views, coloured by life experience and beliefs may prejudice professional judgement when advising patients. In order to guard against this, the disciplined application of moral philosophy, which can be defined as 'the critical evaluation of assumptions and arguments about norms, values, right and wrong, good and bad, and what ought and ought not to be done,'[1] should provide balance.

Although ethical frameworks can help us to debate the best course of action in particular circumstances, it rarely provides 'the answer'. The relative merits of various theories can be contentious. The two main ethical theories are *deontological* and *consequentialist.*

Deontological ethics is based on rights and duties and forms the basis of much religious teaching, in addition to professional codes of practice, such as the General Medical Council's 'Duties of a Doctor'.[2] Consequentialist ethics concerns the effects or consequences of actions and includes utilitarianism, which strives for the greatest good for the majority. Consequentialists may argue, for example, that 'the end justifies the means'.

These theories are not mutually exclusive, but would weight considerations differently.

A further approach to ethical reasoning uses the four principles described by Beauchamp and Childress.[3]

Autonomy (self determination)

The concept of autonomy is highly valued in western society. It is taken to mean the ability of the individual to make decisions about their own life, and relies on informed consent, informed refusal, truth-telling, and confidentiality. An autonomous individual also requires the capacity to understand and weigh information in order to exercise choice.

Non-maleficence (do no harm)

This principle of non-maleficence dates back to the Hippocratic Oath that states that treatment should never be used to injure or wrong the sick. Some procedures may cause harm to a patient and this may or may not be foreseen. Morally, if the harm was unintentional or unforeseen, or the risk judged to be worth taking for the desired benefit, and a standard of due care applied, an act would not be considered to be wrong.

Beneficence (strive to do good)

Beneficence and non-maleficence form a continuum, but medical practice demands more than simply not harming patients; we must positively act to confer benefit on them. This may be at odds with autonomy if a patient decides to reject a doctor's advice, and can lead to paternalistic decision-making.

Justice (fairness, entitlement)

Health care professionals must have due regard for the population at large, for example, by the fair use of resources. The concept of justice can be interpreted as equitable and appropriate treatment to patients in relation to society as a whole.

Ethics in palliative care

Palliative care thrives on good multi-professional teamwork, and this provides the ideal setting for these issues to be debated. Team members will lean towards different theories, and an understanding of this, in addition to a willingness to debate the relative values, will help to achieve the best decision-making with individual patients.

Each theory must be understood, weighted, and applied. For example, the four principles will be in conflict for many complex decisions, and the team must consider the relative merits of each. Key issues relating to nerve blocking and neuromodulation techniques in palliative care, that may entail complex decision-making will include informed consent, resuscitation, withdrawing treatment, carer issues, and resource allocation.

Informed consent

Few would argue that doctors have a duty to give patients all relevant information about their condition and possible treatments. Only by doing this in a way that patients understand (with due regard to clarity, ethnicity, and understanding of individuals), can patients make choices and exert their autonomy. However, doctors vary in what they consider to be relevant. How often does a complication have to occur before patients are warned of it; 1:10, 1:100, 1:1000, 1:10,000? How should such risks be communicated[4–7]? Would warning a patient of a very small risk of a particular procedure cause them harm (*non-maleficence*) or enhance choice (*autonomy*)? The same applies to prescribing medicines beyond their licence—should doctors always inform patients when they do this, or is the information irrelevant and burdensome? Do doctors have a duty to do more than simply give *information* about choices—should they give *advice* (*beneficence*)? Western medicine in recent years has mirrored society's values and prized autonomy very highly, potentially at the expense of other values. The paternalism of medicine in the early part of the last century has been replaced by the 'rights' of patients, epitomized in the UK by the Patients Charter.[8] However, some authors have argued that a doctor's duty is far more complex.[9] Patients may make unwise decisions through fear, denial, misunderstanding, depression, anxiety, and a myriad of other ill-founded reasons. Doctors must work with patients to unravel the decision-making process. Should a doctor ever persuade, or even coerce, a patient to make a decision that the doctor considers to be right (*consequentialism, beneficence, non-maleficence*)? Should patients be given all options even if it means extensive use of resources that could benefit others (*justice*)? How should we weight these principles?

Although few would argue that doctors have a duty to give patients information to reach an informed decision on treatment, when we analyse the principle of informed consent more closely, it raises many more questions. These are all relevant when discussing options for pain management with patients. Our own views may colour the way in which we give information. Experience of the most recent patient who had a successful nerve block, or a serious complication, may colour a doctor's judgement. Some doctors may 'ration' choices in the light of resources, others may advise or even coerce. Self awareness, an understanding of the principles of ethical reasoning, and a healthy discussion within the multi-professional team can help to optimize patient involvement in these difficult decisions.

Resuscitation

Patients with palliative care needs have, by nature of the specialty, an advanced, progressive, and life-threatening disease. Many will have discussed resuscitation issues with family and staff, and come to a decision about their wishes. For others, do not attempt resuscitation (DNAR) orders may be in place on the grounds of futility,[10] without explicit discussion. Discussion with patients may enhance their *autonomy* if there is a real choice to be made, although it runs the risk of maleficence if it raises unrealistic expectations of the process or outcome of resuscitation attempts.

This holds true where it is the disease per se that is causing deterioration and death. However, in some circumstances, the treatment given may cause complications that require resuscitation, such as an intercostal nerve block causing a pneumothorax, or epidural injection resulting in severe hypotension. Although such risks will have been discussed as part of the process of consent, the principle of *non-maleficence* holds that doctors will not wish to cause harm directly to their patients. Due care must be exercised, not only in the choice of procedure for individual patients, but in the facilities available (both suitably trained staff and appropriate equipment). Some procedures can only be performed in an operating theatre with a second anaesthetist, whereas others can be done at the bedside with the help of a health care assistant. Difficulty arises if a patient is too ill to move to an appropriate environment or facilities are not available. In such circumstances, the doctor must work with the patient and family to reach the best possible decision (*beneficence*). Careful risk assessment is mandatory.

Withdrawing treatment

Nerve blocking and neuromodulation techniques rarely prolong life; so ethical dilemmas about the withdrawal of treatment do not need to consider the aspect of potentially shortening life. In this context, withdrawal of treatment is a pragmatic approach to optimum symptom control. As death approaches, the use of indwelling catheters for drug delivery may become unnecessary for some patients. If symptoms can be managed by an alternative means, the nerve block may become superfluous. Clearly it is vital to establish adequate alternative analgesia before taking such a decision. The timing of the termination of a nerve block should be discussed with all members of the caring team, and the patient and family as appropriate. The reason for discontinuation of such treatment should also be explicit, as it may be mis-interpreted as 'giving up on the patient'. A common reason for reviewing a nerve block as death approaches might be that trigger was incident pain that becomes less of a problem as the patient becomes more immobile.

Carer issues

Palliative care practitioners have always considered both the patient and family to be the 'unit of care'. Care is extended to the family and carers throughout the illness and into bereavement. It is considered to be good practice that family members are involved in decision-making and care planning throughout, with the consent of the patient. The doctor's prime concern should be to the patient,[2] and this extends to patients who are no longer competent to make their own decisions, when the doctor must act in their 'best interests'. This is an example of *beneficence,* and includes collecting evidence of the patient's prior wishes from friends, family members, or advance directives. This is not contentious unless there is a conflict of views between the patient and family or professional carers. However, patients' choices may have detrimental effects on others. No one is a completely *autonomous* individual, as we all rely on others for aspects of our well-being. A patient's *autonomy* may be in conflict with the *autonomy* of a relative or professional carer; for example, a patient with extensive nursing needs, who was to be cared for in the family home, will need the support of family members and potential alterations to the house. In these situations, the team must decide whether the best course of action is 'the best outcome for the majority' (*consequentialist/utilitarian*) or the prime duty of care to the patient (*deontology*).

Resource allocation

No doctor can treat a patient in isolation from other pressures on resources, such as time, equipment, finance, or beds. The prime duty of care to the patient must be balanced with the concept of distributive *justice*. This is relevant in the choice of drugs and procedures offered to patients that must be chosen wisely, with due regard to alternatives that may produce equivalent results.

Closing remarks

This chapter provides a framework for clinicians working within multi-professional teams to base complex decision-making within a moral structure. This goes some way to guarding against decisions based on prejudice or on the experience of memorable patients who may have had good or bad outcomes. Nerve blocking and neuromodulation techniques have a clear place within pain management strategies in palliative care and should be considered early for patients whose pain is not well managed by other means.

Further reading

Gillon R (1996). *Philosophical medical ethics*. John Wiley & Sons, Chichester, UK.

Beauchamp TL and Childress JF (1994). *Principles of biomedical ethics*. Oxford University Press, Oxford.

References

1. Raphael DD (1981). *Moral philosophy*. Oxford University Press, Oxford.
2. General Medical Council (1998). *Good medical practice*. General Medical Council, London.
3. Beauchamp TL and Childress JF (1994). *Principles of biomedical ethics*. Oxford University Press, Oxford.
4. Edwards A (2003). Communicating risks. *Br Med J* **327**:691–2.
5. Godolphin W (2003). The role of risk communication in shared decision making. *Br Med J* **327**:692–3.
6. Thornton H (2003). Patients' understanding of risk. *Br Med J* **327**:693-4.
7. Sedgewick P and Hall A (2003). Teaching medical students and doctors how to communicate risk. *Br Med J* **327**:694–5.
8. The stationery office, London. Department of Health (1996). The patients' charter and you, a charter for England.
9. Marzuk PM (1985). The right kind of paternalism. *New Eng J Med* **313**(23):1474–6.
10. National Council for Hospice and Specialist Palliative Care Services (2002). Ethical decision making in palliative care: cardiopulmonary resuscitation (CPR) for people who are terminally ill. NCHSPCS, London.

Index

Page numbers in *italic* indicate figures and tables.